2022-23 Peripheral PHARMACIST

Jeanine P. Abrons, PharmD, MS, FAPhA

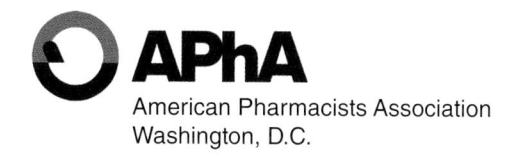

APhA
American Pharmacists Association
Washington, D.C.

Senior Director, Books and Digital Publishing: Eleanore Tapscott
Editorial Director: Jesse Vineyard
Production Editor: Brittany Williams
Editorial Services: Circle Graphics
Cover Design: Michelle I. Powell, APhA Integrated Design and Production

©2022 by the American Pharmacists Association
APhA was founded in 1852 as the American Pharmaceutical Association

Published by the American Pharmacists Association
2215 Constitution Avenue, NW
Washington, DC 20037-2985
www.pharmacist.com
www.pharmacylibrary.com

All rights reserved

No part of this publication may be reproduced, stored in a retrieval system, or transmitted in any form or by any means, electronic, mechanical, photocopying, recording, or otherwise, without written permission from the publisher.

To comment on this book by e-mail, send your message to the publisher at *aphabooks@aphanet.org*.

Library of Congress Cataloging-in-Publication Data available upon request.

How to Order This Book

Online: www.pharmacist.com/shop
By phone: 800-878-0729 (770-280-0085 from outside the United States)
VISA®, MasterCard®, and American Express® cards accepted.

Contents

CARDIOLOGY
Hypertension Management 1
Atherosclerotic Cardiovascular Disease (ASCVD) Risk......................... 5
Lipid Goals Based Upon Level of Risk—AACE Guidelines 8
Treating LDL-C to Goal in Patients with Diabetes 8
Statin Intensity-Based ASCVD Risk in Patients with Diabetes................. 9
Moderate and High-Intensity Statin Therapy..................................... 9
Cholesterol Management: Use of Drug Classes Other than Statins............. 10
Direct Oral Anticoagulants **(NEW UPDATES)** 12
Transitioning from Injectable Anticoagulants to Direct-Acting
  Oral Anticoagulants (DOACs)... 16
Injectable Anticoagulants 18
Perioperative Management of Direct Oral Anticoagulants 20
Common Warfarin Drug Interactions.. 21
Warfarin Dosing Principles... 22
Alterations to Warfarin Dose Maintenance Therapy 24
ACLS Drugs by Arrhythmia Type or Condition 26

ENDOCRINOLOGY
Diabetes Treatment Guidelines.. 27
Patient-Centered Glycemic Collaborative Care in the Management
  in Type 2 Diabetes Decision Cycle 28
Associated Goals for Adults with Diabetes **(NEW)** 29
Type 2 Diabetes: Glycemic Control Approaches 30
Medications for Type 2 Diabetes 32
Insulin and Insulin Analogues... 34

RESPIRATORY
Asthma: Definition & Diagnosis—Based on the 2021 GINA Guidelines **(NEW)** .. 35
Asthma: Assessment of Level of Control—Based on the 2021 GINA
  Guidelines **(NEW)** 36
Initial Asthma Treatment Steps and Recommended Options for Adults
  and Adolescents Based on the 2021 GINA Guidelines **(NEW)** 37
Selecting Initial Controller Treatment in Children Ages 6 to 11 with
  a Diagnosis of Asthma—Based on the 2021 GINA Guidelines **(NEW)** 38
Personalized Asthma Management Continuous Cycle......................... 38
Suggested Low, Medium, and High Dosing of Inhaled Corticosteroids
  in Asthma... 39
Assessment of Airflow Limitation/Symptoms in Chronic Obstructive
  Pulmonary Disease (COPD) **(NEW)**.. 40
Assessment to Determine ABCD Groups in Chronic Obstructive
  Pulmonary Disease (COPD) **(NEW)** 41
Initial Therapies Based on Symptom Severity/Exacerbation Risk for COPD 42
COPD Follow-Up 43
COPD Exacerbation Management (Severe but not Life-Threatening)........... 43
COVID-19 in Patients with COPD 44
Common Maintenance Medications Used in COPD 44

Contents

INFECTIOUS DISEASES
Testing for COVID-19 **(NEW)** 46
Collecting, Handling, and Testing of Clinical Specimens for COVID-19 **(NEW)** 47
Collecting Anterior Nasal Swab and Nasal Mid-Turbinate Specimens
for COVID-19 Testing 48
Community-Acquired Pneumonia (CAP) Management 49
Treatment of Community-Acquired Pneumonia (CAP) 50
Hospital-Acquired Pneumonia (HAP) Management 51
Aminoglycosides: Traditional Considerations and Dosing in Adults............... 53
Aminoglycosides: Single Daily Dosing 54
Vancomycin: Considerations and Dosing in Adults............................. 55
Vancomycin: General Information and Dosing (PO/IV) for *C. difficile* Colitis 56
Sample Antimicrobial Coverage... 57
Gram Stain Interpretation: GRAM + RESULT 61
Gram Stain Interpretation: GRAM − RESULT 62
Consideration of When to Draw Cultures vs. Start Antibiotics
in the Emergency Department (ED) **(NEW)** 63
Consider When to & Whether to Draw a Culture 64
Examples of Considerations by Culture Type 64

SPECIAL POPULATIONS
Pediatric
Information for Pharmacists for Parents During COVID-19..................... 65
Usual Pediatric Dosages of Common Over-the-Counter (OTC) Medications 66
Pediatric Commercially Available Dosage Forms and Doses/
Concentrations of Analgesics 67
Pediatric Commercially Available Dosage Forms and Doses/
Concentrations of Antihistamines... 68
Pediatric Commercially Available Dosage Forms and Doses for Gastrointestinal
or Motion Sickness Purposes **(NEW)** 70
Use of Creams in Pediatric Populations 71
Pediatric Measurements **(NEW)** 71
Geriatric
Inappropriate Medications in Older Adults 72
Women's Health
Pregnancy and Lactation Resources: Medication-Related Resources 74
Pregnancy Risk Classifications... 75
Safe and Unsafe Use of OTC Medications during Pregnancy -
Various Conditions 76
Safe and Unsafe Use of OTC Medications during Pregnancy -
Gastrointestinal Medications.. 77

IMMUNIZATIONS **(UPDATED ANNUALLY)**
Immunization Schedule for Children and Adolescent Ages 18 Years or Younger 78
Immunizations by Age for First Year of Life 82
2021 Recommended Immunizations for Children from Birth Through 6 Years Old 83
Travel Immunization and Travel Health Card **(NEW ADDITIONS)** 84

Contents

CALCULATIONS/CONVERSIONS/PATIENT ASSESSMENT & MONITORING
Conversions
Conversions.. 90
Weights and Measures 91
Apothecary Equivalents... 92
Opioid Conversions... 93
Systemic Corticosteroid Conversions.................................... 94
Calculations
How to Work Up a Patient (*Inpatient/Ambulatory Care*) 95
Sample Patient Workup Card for Use In Patient Care................................ 100
Acid and Base Imbalances—An Overview and Implications for the Pharmacist 104
Acid–Base Disorders—The Basics 105
Creatinine Clearance Calculations 107
Patient Assessment and Monitoring
Target Serum Concentrations for Selected Drugs 108

SPECIFIC DISEASE STATE MANAGEMENT
Psychiatry Guidelines... 109
Psychiatric Medications 110
Nutrition 111
Electrolyte & Mineral Requirements—Influences of Needs 116
Chronic Kidney Disease.. 117
Pain Management.. 120
Co-Prescribing Naloxone for Outpatient Settings.................. 121
Similarities and Differences Between Naloxone Formulations.................... 122
Recommending Naloxone to a Patient.................................. 123
Veterinary Medicine Information **(NEW)**........................... 125
Transplant Medications 126

MISCELLANEOUS
Free Quality Online Resources.. 131
National Clinical Guidelines 132
Clinically Significant Drug Interactions 134
Medications with Adverse Withdrawal Effects from Abrupt Discontinuation........ 135
FASTHUG-MAIDENS: Approach to Identifying Drug-Related Problems (DRPs)
& Aspects of Critical Care for Intensive Care Units (ICU) Pharmacists 138
Pharmacy Mnemonics and Memory Aids: Dosing/Drug Names and Interactions.... 140
Diversity, Equity, Inclusion, Accessibility, Bias, and Cultural Awareness **(NEW)**.... 141

INTEGRATIVE MEDICINE
Herbal or Botanical Therapies.. 149
Herbal or Botanical Medicine 152
Basics of Medical Cannabis... 161
FDA-Approved Medical Cannabis Products........................... 162
Possible Uses of Medical Cannabis 162
Pharmacology Basics of Medical Cannabis........................... 163
Dosing/Side Effects of Medical Cannabis.............................. 163
Medical Cannabis & Examples of Drug Interactions 164
Medical Cannabis: Evidence and Special Populations 164
Cannabidiol (CBD): A Naturally Occurring Cannabinoid Found in Cannabis 165

COUNSELING AND STANDARDS OF CARE
Motivational Interviewing Techniques 166
Empathic Communication Skills for Pharmacists 167
Delivering Bad News.. 168
NURSE Acronym for Responding to Emotions...................... 169
Differentiating Empathy Versus Sympathy............................ 170
Common Problematic Phrases in Communication to Avoid..................... 171
Pharmacists' Patient Care Process....................................... 172
Choosing Your Counseling Points.. 174

v

Call for Ideas

Submit ideas for new cards in future editions of the *Peripheral Brain*. Send your ideas to aphabooks@aphanet.org. Thanks!

Please let us know the most useful content or additional areas that you'd like to see in the future to further increase the value of this product.

Contributors

AUTHORS

BEN MISKLE, PharmD
University of Iowa College of Pharmacy
Iowa City, Iowa

LOC NGUYEN, PharmD
Consultant Pharmacist
Houston, Texas

HALEY MORRISON, PharmD
CVS Pharmacy
Cedar Falls, Iowa

SHUSHANNA GALSTYAN, PharmD
Pharmacist
Pasadena, California

JEANINE P. ABRONS, PharmD, MS
Clinical Associate Professor/Director of
  Student Pharmacists International Activities/
  Co-Director UI Mobile Clinics
University of Iowa College of Pharmacy
Iowa City, Iowa

SWATHI VARANASI, PharmD
Integrative Health Pharmacist
Los Angeles, California

LANE NGUYEN, PharmD, BCPPS
Clinical Pharmacy Specialist,
  Pediatric Critical Care Medicine
Memorial Sloan Kettering Cancer Center
New York, New York

ELISHA ANDREAS, PharmD, MPH
Pharmacist
Hartig Drug
Iowa City, Iowa

JANAN SARWAR, PharmD
CEO, Global Bookshelves International
CCO, The Happy PharmD
Medical Program Manager, CMEOutfitters
Louisville, Kentucky

EMILY PAULUS, PharmD Candidate 2022
University of Iowa College of Pharmacy
Iowa City, Iowa

JENNA BLUNT, PharmD, BCPS
Clinical Pharmacy Specialist
MercyOne
Des Moines, Iowa

ERIKA BETHHAUSER, PharmD
PGY-1 Pharmacy Resident
Veterans Affairs Central Iowa Health Care System
Des Moines, Iowa

MICHAEL J. PARISI MERCADO, PharmD, MPH
PGY1 Pharmacy (Acute Care Focus) Resident
Froedtert & the Medical College of Wisconsin
Milwaukee, Wisconsin

KASHELLE LOCKMAN, PharmD
Clinical Assistant Professor
University of Iowa College of Pharmacy
Iowa City, Iowa

THEODORE NGUYEN, PharmD, BCPS
Pharmacist
Los Angeles County Department of Mental Health
Los Angeles, California

MARK BOTTI, PharmD, BCPPS, AE-C
Pharmacist
Albany Medical Center
Albany, New York

CRYSTAL McELHOSE, PharmD, MPH
PGY-1 Resident
Allen Hospital
Waterloo, Iowa

THOMAS ROBERTS, PharmD
PGY1 Pharmacy Resident
Veterans Affairs Central Iowa Health Care System
Des Moines, Iowa

ASHLEY BEHRENS, PharmD, BCPS
Clinical Pharmacist
Veterans Affairs Central Iowa Health Care System
Des Moines, Iowa

STEVEN HONG, PharmD
Pharmacist
Iowa City, Iowa

ANH LUONG, PharmD
Pharmacist
Greene County Hospital
Jefferson, Iowa

KELLY SHEA, PharmD
Clinical Staff Pharmacist
Unity Point
Des Moines, Iowa

VERN DUBA, MA
Clinical Assistant Professor
University of Iowa College of Pharmacy
Iowa City, Iowa

NICOLE BUCCI, PharmD
Pharmacist
Albany Medical Center
Albany, New York

APRYL JACOBS, PharmD, BCPS
Decentralized Pharmacists
St. Peter's Hospital
Albany, New York

SHAWN PHILLIPS, PharmD, BCPS
Pharmacist
St. Peter's Medical Center
Albany, New York

Contributors

ERICA MACEIRA, PharmD, BCPS, CACP
Associate Director of Pharmacy – Clinical Services
Renal/Pancreas Transplant Pharmacist
Pharmacy Residency Director
Intern Coordinator
Albany Medical Center
Albany, New York

MOLLY HENRY, PharmD
Solid Organ Transplant Clinical Pharmacist
University of Nebraska Medical Center
Omaha, Nebraska

JOANNA RUSCH, PharmD
Pharmacist
Ready Meds Pharmacy
Renton, WA

BRYAN PINCKNEY WHITE, PharmD, BCPS
Infectious Diseases Clinical Pharmacist
Oklahoma University Medical Center
Oklahoma City, OKlahoma

ANGELA WOJTCZAK, PharmD
Clinical Pharmacy Specialist at Rush University Medical Center
Northbrook, IL

MARISSA RUPALO, PharmD Candidate 2022
University of Iowa College of Pharmacy
Iowa City, Iowa

EMMA PIEHL, PharmD Candidate 2022
University of Iowa College of Pharmacy
Iowa City, Iowa

Reviewers

BRIGID K. GROVES, PharmD, MS
Senior Director, Practice and Professional Affairs
American Pharmacists Association
Washington, D.C.

PARIA SANATY ZADEH, PharmD
Associate Director, Practice and Science Programs
American Pharmacists Association
Washington, D.C

HAILEY MOOK, PharmD
Executive Resident, Education
American Pharmacists Association

JERI SIAS, PharmD, MPH
Clinical Professor
University of Texas at El Paso School of Pharmacy
El Paso, TX

Acknowledgments

The editor and publisher gratefully acknowledge Jennifer Cerulli, PharmD, BCPS, and Renée Ahrens Thomas, PharmD, MBA, for their help in selecting the contents of previous editions; and Jennifer L. Adams, PharmD, EdD, and Keith D. Marciniak, BSPharm, who developed the concept of reference cards in an APhA resource that preceded *Peripheral Brain for the Pharmacist*. The editor and publisher gratefully recognize Alecia Heh for her involvement in previous versions of diabetes-related pages, Ben Lomaestro for his previous work with the infectious disease–related cards, and Eric P. Boateng for his work on the Medications with Adverse Withdrawal Effects from Abrupt Discontinuation pages.

Additional thanks and acknowledgment to the following former authors for their contributions: Sara E. Dugan, PharmD, BCPP, BCPS; Jasmine Mangrum, PharmD, MPH; Jessica Carswell, PharmD; Rebecca Petrik, PharmD; Brittany Hayes, BS, RRT, RCP, PharmD; Adrienne Rouiller, PharmD; Vassilia Sidera, PharmD; Anastasia Lundt, PharmD; and Breanna Sunderman, PharmD. This book is dedicated to my students, both past and current, who inspire me to continue to think about what is relevant to pharmacy practice; and to my children, Linus and Violet, my husband, Ron; and my family, who inspire me to always learn more and to provide resources to enhance learning and patient care.

Hypertension Management

High Blood Pressure Guideline Summary: The 2017 Guideline for the Prevention, Detection, Evaluation, & Management of High Blood Pressure in Adults represents an update of the Joint National Committee (JNC) guidelines from 2003. The guidelines include information from studies on related risk of cardiovascular disease (CVD) & monitoring, & include thresholds to start drug treatment & goals.

Classifying High Blood Pressure (BP) in Adults

CATEGORY	SYSTOLIC Blood Pressure (SBP) in mmHg		DIASTOLIC Blood Pressure (DBP) in mmHg
Normal	< 120	AND	< 80
Elevated	120 to 129	AND	< 80
Hypertension (HTN) • Stage 1 • Stage 2	130 to 139 ≥ 140	OR OR	80 to 89 ≥ 90

Patient with high SBP & DBP in 2 categories: select the higher category.
Caution: BP is based on an average of ≥ 2 readings taken on ≥ 2 occasions.
BP measurements in clinical trial may not represent typical level of care & patient motivation.

Use of CVD Risk Estimation* and Blood Pressure Threshold to Guide Drug Treatment	
Use of BP-lowering medications are recommended for:	
Stage 1 Hypertension: *130 to 139/80 to 89 mmHg*	• ASCVD or 10-year CVD risk ≥ 10% • No ASCVD and 10-year CVD risk < 10% ○ If BP not at goal three to six months following non-pharmacologic therapy
Stage 2 Hypertension: *≥ 140/≥ 90 mmHg*	• **BP at goal with current therapy/regimen:** reassess every three to six months • **BP not at goal with current therapy/regimen:** assess adherence & consider therapy intensification
Initial Monotherapy Versus Initial Combination Drug Therapy	

- ***Stage 1 hypertension (HTN) & BP goal < 130/80 mmHg:***
  Start 1 antihypertensive drug. Titrate dose & sequentially add other agents to achieve BP target.
- ***Stage 2 hypertension & average BP > 20/10 mmHg above target:***
  Start 2 first-line agents of different classes, either as separate agents or in fixed-dose combination.

Initial Medication Options

- ***First-line agents:*** ACE or ARB, thiazide diuretics, & CCB

*Notes: *ACC/AHA Risk Estimator Plus: http://tools.acc.org/ASCVD-Risk-Estimator-Plus/ (Accessed 2021); ASCVD was defined as a first congenital heart disease death, nonfatal myocardial infarction or nonfatal stroke. ASCVD = atherosclerotic cardiovascular disease; ACE = angiotensin conversion enzyme inhibitor; ARB = angiotensin receptor blocker; CCB = calcium channel blocker.*

Reference: https://www.acc.org/latest-in-cardiology/articles/2021/06/21/13/05/new-guidance-on-bp-management-in-low-risk-adults-with-stage-1-htn (Accessed November 2021)

Hypertension Management *(continued)*

Considerations in Care – Management of High Blood Pressure

CONSIDERATION	DESCRIPTION	
Blood Pressure Management	• Accurate management is critical. • Consider out-of-office & self-monitoring to confirm & titrate medications. • Measurement values may vary depending on time & location taken.	
Screen/Manage Other CVD Risk Factors	• Smoking; diabetes; dyslipidemia; weight; low fitness; poor diet; stress; sleep apnea • Testing	
	BASIC testing	Complete blood count; fasting blood glucose; lipid profile; serum creatinine with estimated glomerular filtration rate (eGFR); serum electrolytes (K^+; Na^{2+}; Ca^{2+}); thyroid-stimulating hormone (TSH); urinalysis; electrocardiogram
	OPTIONAL testing	Echocardiogram; uric acid; urine albumin to creatinine ratio
Screen for Secondary Causes of Hypertension (HTN)	• Screen for common secondary causes with new-onset or uncontrolled hypertension. • If more specific clinical symptoms are present, consider uncommon secondary causes.	
	COMMON Causes to prompt need to screen for secondary causes of hypertension	
	• Primary aldosteronism (elevated aldosterone/renin ratio) • CKD (chronic kidney disease) (eGFR < 60 mL/min/1.73 m^2) • Renal artery stenosis (young female, known atherosclerotic disease, worsening kidney function) • Obstructive sleep apnea (snoring, witnessed apnea, excessive daytime sleepiness)	• Abrupt onset • Age < 30 • Drug resistant/induced: uncontrolled BP after treatment with ≥ 3 antihypertensives • Excessive target organ damage (e.g., cerebral vascular disease; retinopathy; left ventricular hypertrophy, heart failure [HF] with preserved ejection fraction [EF] or with reserved EF; coronary artery disease [CAD]; chronic kidney disease; peripheral artery disease; albuminuria) • OR onset of diastolic HTN in older adults • OR unprovoked or excessive hypokalemia
	UNCOMMON Causes	
	(< 1%)	• Acromegaly • Aortic coarctation • Congenital adrenal hyperplasia • Mineralocorticoid excess syndrome (not primary aldosteronism) • Cushing syndrome • Hypo-hyperthyroidism or primary hyperparathyroidism • Phenochromocytoma/paraganglioma
Follow-up	**ADULT PATIENT GROUP**	**FREQUENCY OF FOLLOW-UP**
	Low risk with elevated BP or stage 1 HTN with ASCVD risk < 10%	Repeat BP after 3 to 6 months of non-pharmacological therapy
	Stage 1 HTN & high ASCVD risk (≥ 10% 10-year ASCVD risk)	Repeat BP after 1 month of non-pharmacologic & antihypertensive drug therapy
	Stage 2 HTN	Evaluate by primary care provider (PCP) within 1 month of diagnosis; treat with combo of non-pharmacologic & 2 antihypertensive drugs from different classes; repeat evaluation in 1 month
	Very high average BP (systolic ≥ 160 mmHg or diastolic ≥ 100 mmHg)	Evaluate promptly; monitor carefully & adjust dose upward as needed
	Normal BP	Repeat BP evaluation annually

Hypertension Management *(continued)*

Oral Antihypertensives PRIMARY Agents

Medication Class	Drug	General Notes
Thiazide or thiazide-type diuretics	• Chlorthalidone • Idapamide • Hydrochlorothiazide • Metolazone	• Chlorthalidone preferred (*cardiovascular [CVD] reduction & prolonged half-life*) • Monitor Na^{2+} (hyponatremia), K^+ (hypokalemia), Ca^{2+}, & uric acid • History of acute gout: use caution unless already on uric acid–lowering drug
Angiotensin Converting Enzyme (ACE) inhibitors	• Benazepril • Captopril • Enalapril • Fosinopril • Lisinopril • Moexipril • Perindopril • Quinapril • Ramipril • Trandolapril	• Don't use with ARBs or direct renin inhibitor; history of angioedema on ACE inhibitors • Risk of hyperkalemia with CKD*, K^+-sparing diuretics, or K^+ supplements • Acute renal failure risk in patients with severe bilateral renal artery stenosis • Avoid if pregnant
Angiotensin Receptor Blockers (ARBs)	• Azilsartan • Candesartan • Eprosartan • Irbesartan • Losartan • Olmesartan • Telmisartan • Valsartan	• Don't use with ACE inhibitors or direct renin inhibitor; history of angioedema on ARBs • If angioedema occurred with ACE inhibitor: ARB can be used 6 weeks after stopping ACE inhibitor • Risks of hyperkalemia, acute renal failure, and pregnancy are similar if not same to those for ACE inhibitors
Calcium Channel Blockers (CCB)	• Amlodipine • Felodipine • Isradipine • Nicardipine Sustained Release (SR) • Nifedipine Long Acting (LA) • Nisoldipine	• Avoid use if: heart failure with reduced ejection fraction (HFrEF); if required, use amlodipine or felodipine • Associated with pedal edema (dose-related)
Non-dihydropyridine CCB	• Diltiazem Extended Release (ER) • Verapamil Immediate Release (IR) • Verapamil SR • Verapamil-delayed onset ER	• Routine use with beta blockers should be avoided (risk of bradycardia & heart block) • Don't use if: HFrEF

Hypertension Management *(continued)*

Oral Antihypertensives SECONDARY Agents

Medication Class	Drug	General Notes
Diuretics		
Loop	• Bumetanide • Furosemide • Torsemide	• Preferred if: symptomatic heart failure (HF) • Preferred over thiazides if: moderate to severe CKD *(GFR < 30 mL/min)*
Potassium-sparing	• Amiloride • Triametene	• Monotherapy & minimally effective • If hypokalemia on thiazide monotherapy, can add potassium-sparing diuretic to the thiazide diuretic • Avoid if: significant CKD (GFR < 45 mL/min)
Aldosterone antagonists	• Eplerenone • Spironolactone	• Preferred if: resistant hypertension/primary aldosteronism • Spironolactone: higher risk of gynecomastia/impotence • Avoid use with: K$^+$ supplements, K$^+$-sparing diuretics, or significant renal dysfunction • Eplerenone often requires twice-daily dosing
Beta-Blockers		
Cardioselective	• Atenolol • Betaxolol • Bisoprolol • Metoprolol tartrate • Metoprolol succinate	• Not first line unless ischemic heart disease (IHD) or HF • Preferred if: bronchospastic airway disease • If HFrEF, bisoprolol & metoprolol succinate preferred • Avoid stopping abruptly
Cardioselective/vasodilatory	• Nebivolol	• Avoid stopping abruptly
Non-cardioselective	• Nadolol • Propranolol IR* • Propranolol Long Acting (LA)	• Avoid in reactive airways disease • Avoid stopping abruptly
Intrinsic sympathomimetic	• Acebutolol • Penbutolol • Pindolol	• Avoid, especially in IHD or HF • Avoid stopping abruptly
Alpha/beta-receptor	• Carvedilol • Carvedilol phosphate • Labetalol	• If HFrEF: Carvedilol preferred • Avoid stopping abruptly
Direct renin inhibitor	• Aliskiren	• Don't use with: ACE inhibitors or ARBs • Risk of hyperkalemia with: CKD &/or on K$^+$-sparing drugs/supplements • If severe bilateral renal artery stenosis, risk of acute renal failure • Avoid in pregnancy
Alpha-1 blockers	• Doxazosin • Prazosin • Terazosin	• Associated with orthostatic hypotension, especially in older adults • Second-line if: patient has benign prostatic hyperplasia (BPH)
Centrally acting drugs	• Clonidine oral & patch • Methyldopa • Guanfacine	• Last line: central nervous system (CNS) adverse effects • Clonidine: taper to avoid rebound hypertension & avoid stopping abruptly (risk of hypertensive crisis)
Direct vasodilators	• Hydralazine • Minoxidil	• Associated with sodium/water retention & reflex tachycardia: use with a diuretic & beta blocker • High doses of hydralazine: associated with lupus-like syndrome • Minoxidil: hirsutism & pericardial effusion risks; use loop diuretic

*Note: * = IR*

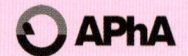

Atherosclerotic Cardiovascular Disease (ASCVD) Risk

ASCVD Risk Estimation Calculator:
http://tools.acc.org/ascvd-risk-estimator-plus/#!/calculate/estimate/ (Accessed 2021)

Other Potential Scoring Systems for Cardiovascular Risk

Scoring System	Notes on Scoring System	Calculator or Additional Information Available
Multi-Ethnic Study of Atherosclerosis (MESA)	• Most appropriate for patients 45 to 85 years old & in the following racial/ethnic groups: White, Asian (of Chinese descent), African American, or Hispanic • Incorporates coronary artery calcium	• https://mesa-nhlbi.org/MESACHDRisk/MesaRiskScore/RiskScore.aspx • https://pubmed.ncbi.nlm.nih.gov/34167645/
Reynolds Risk Score for Cardiovascular Risk	• For women > 45 years old • Largely white healthcare professionals enrolled in clinical trials • Includes inflammatory marker in score	• http://www.reynoldsriskscore.org
UK Prospective Diabetes Study (UKPDS) Risk	• Scoring system for type 2 diabetes	• https://www.dtu.ox.ac.uk/riskengine/

Note: All websites accessed 2021.

Risk Factors for Atherosclerotic Cardiovascular Disease

Major Risk Factors	Other (Additional or Nontraditional)
• ↑ Age • ↑ Serum cholesterol • ↑ Non-HDL • ↑ LDL-C • Low HDL-C • Diabetes mellitus • Hypertension • Chronic kidney disease • Tobacco use • Family history of premature ASCVD	• Obesity/abdominal obesity • Family history of hyperlipidemia • ↑ small, dense LDL-C • ↑ Apo-lipoprotein B • ↑ LDL particle concentration • Fasting/postprandial hypertriglyeridemia • PCOS • Dyslipidemic triad* • ↑ Lipoprotein (a) • ↑ Clotting factors • ↑ Inflammatory markers (hsCRP; Lp-PLA$_2$)

*Notes: HDL = high-density lipoprotein; LDL = low-density lipoprotein; C = cholesterol; PCOS = polycystic ovarian syndrome; hsCRP = high sensitive C-reactive protein; Lp-PLA$_2$ = lipoprotein-associated phospholipase. * = hypertriglyceridemia (triglycerides >150 mg/dL); low high-density lipoprotein cholesterol (HDL-C; ≤ 35 mg/dL); and small, dense low-density lipoprotein particles.*

Reference: Modified from Table 6 – Clinical Practice Guidelines for Managing Dyslipidemia & Prevention of CVD, Endocr Pract. 2017;23(Suppl 2) 17 Copyright © 2017 AACE; Arnett DK, Blumenthal RS, Albert MA, et al. 2019 ACC/AHA guideline on the primary prevention of cardiovascular disease: a report of the American College of Cardiology/American Heart Association Task Force on Clinical Practice Guidelines. Journal of the American College of Cardiology. 2019;74(10):e177–232

Atherosclerotic Cardiovascular Disease (ASCVD) Risk (continued)

Steps to Determine Management Strategy to Reduce Lipids and Risk of Atherosclerotic Cardiovascular Disease

Step #	Overall Step	Description of Step
1	Determine ASCVD risk.	Use a scoring system for cardiovascular risk, determine if the patient does or does not have clinical ASCVD, &/or measure a coronary artery calcium score.
2	Encourage a healthy lifestyle.	• Individualize lifestyle modifications to each patient. • May include smoking cessation, diet modification, physical activity, & weight ↓ to target an optimal weight.
3	Consider medications.	• Discuss selection of lipid-lowering medications including benefit/risk/cost analysis. • As ASCVD risk ↑ benefits of evidence-based lipid-lowering medications also ↑.
4	If treatment favors lipid-lowering medications, use evidence-based medicine. (Assess ASCVD risk by age group & emphasize adherence to healthy lifestyle.)	**Primary Prevention** | Patient Factor	Recommendation
---	---
LDL-C ≥ 190 mg/dL	No risk assessment; use high-intensity statin
Diabetes & age 40 to 75 years old:	• Moderate-intensity statin • Risk assessment to consider high-intensity statin
Age 0 to 19 years old	• Lifestyle modifications to ↓ ASCVD risk • With diagnosis of familial hypercholesterolemia: statin
Age 20 to 39 years old	• Lifetime risk estimation • Consider statin if family history (FH) or premature ASCVD & LDL-C ≥ 160 mg/dL
Age 40 to 75 years old without diabetes and LDL 70 to 18mg/dL	• For all risk levels, discuss risk ↓ • Risk < 5 %: emphasize lifestyle to ↓ risk factors • Risk 5 to < 7.5%: may + moderate intensity statin • Risk ≥ 7.5 to < 20%: may + moderate intensity statin to ↓ LDL-C by 30 to 49% • ≥ 20%, + statin to ↓ LDL-C by ≥ 50%
Age > 75 years old	Clinical assessment & risk discussion | **Secondary Prevention** (refer to page 8 for definitions) | ASCVD not at very high risk	Very high risk ASCVD
---	---

• For age ≤ 75 years old, use high-intensity statin with a goal LDL-C ↓ of ≥ 50%:
  ○ If high-intensity statin not tolerated, use moderate-intensity statin
  ○ On max statin therapy & LDL-C ≥ 70 mg/dL + may add ezetimibe
• For age > 75 years old: reasonable to initiate moderate- or high-intensity statin OR continuation of high-intensity statin is reasonable
	• Use high-intensity or maximal statin:
	  ○ If on max statin & LDL-C ≥ 70 mg/dL + may add ezetimibe
	  ○ If PCS9-I is considered, add ezetimibe to max statin before + PCSK9-I
	  ○ If on max LDL-C ↓ therapy & LDL-C ≥ 70 mg/dL or non-HDL-C ≥ 100 mg/dL may + PCSK9-I	

5	Regularly reassess.	Frequently evaluate patient goals for ASCVD risk ↓, medication tolerability/affordability, and treatment plans.

Note: LDL-C = low-density lipoprotein cholesterol; non-HDL = non-high-density lipoprotein; PCSK9-I = proprotein convertase subtilisin/kexin type 9 serine protease inhibitor.

References: Table modified from: Arnett DK, Blumenthal RS, Albert MA, et al. 2019 ACC/AHA guideline on the primary prevention of cardiovascular disease: a report of the American College of Cardiology/American Heart Association Task Force on Clinical Practice Guidelines. Journal of the American College of Cardiology. 2019; 74(10):e177–232; Figure 1: Secondary Prevention in Patients with Clinical ASCVD & Figure 2: Primary Prevention in Grundy SM, Stone NJ, Bailey AL, Beam C, Birtcher KK et al. 2018–AHA/ACC/AACVPR/AAPA/ABC/ACPM/ADA/AGS/APhA/ASPC/NLA/PCNA Guideline on the Management of Blood Cholesterol. A Report to the American College of Cardiology/American Heart Association Task Force on Clinical Practice Guidelines. Circulation. 2018. Available at: https://www.ahajournals.org/doi/abs/10.1161/CIR.0000000000000625 (Accessed November 2021)

Atherosclerotic Cardiovascular Disease (ASCVD) Risk *(continued)*

Process of Evaluating a Patient Prior to Initiation of a Statin:

Initial evaluation prior to statin initiation:
- Fasting lipid panel
- Alanine aminotransferase
- Creatinine Kinase (CK) [If indicated]
- Hemoglobin A1c [If diabetes status unknown]
- Consider evaluation for other secondary causes or conditions that may influence statin safety

→

Treat Laboratory Abnormalities
- Triglycerides ≥ 500 mg/dL
- LDL-C ≥ 190 mg/dL
- Unexplained ALT ≥ 3x the Upper Limit of Normal (ULN)

Other Biomarker Monitoring with Cholesterol Management:

Biomarker	Notes
Coronary artery calcium (CAC)	• Consider monitoring if risk decision is unknown • Interpretation: **CAC Value 0** — Lower risk; consider no statin, unless diabetic, family history (FH) of premature coronary heart disease (CHD), or cigarette smoker **CAC Value 1 to 99** — Favors statin use (especially after age 55) **CAC Value 100+ &/or ≥ 75th percentile** — Initiate statin therapy
High-sensitivity C-reactive protein (Hs-CRP)	• Inflammatory marker • Elevation ≥ 2 mg/dL • Measure with persistently elevated triglycerides (TG) ≥ 175 mg/dL
Ankle-brachial index (ABI)	• Ratio of blood pressure (BP) at the ankle to BP in the brachium • Compared to arm, ↓ BP in the leg suggests blocked artery secondary to peripheral artery disease (PAD) • Measure with persistently elevated TG ≥ 175 mg/dL
Lipoprotein A	• Relative indicator for measurement = FH of premature atherosclerotic coronary artery disease (ASCVD) • Measure with persistently elevated triglycerides (TG) ≥ 175 mg/dL

Reference: Based on recommendations from Grundy SM, Stone NJ, Bailey AL, Beam C, Birtcher KK et al. 2018–AHA/ACC/AACVPR/AAPA/ACPM/ADA/AGS/AphA/ASPC/NLA/PCNA Guideline on the Management of Blood Cholesterol. A Report to the American College of Cardiology/American Heart Association Task Force on Clinical Practice Guidelines. Circulation, 2018. Available at: https://www.ahajournals.org/doi/abs/10.1161/CIR.0000000000000625 (Accessed November 2021)

Lipid Goals Based Upon Level of Risk—AACE Guidelines

Level of Risk	Risk Factors/10-year Risk	Treatment Goals (In mg/dL)
Extreme	• Progressive ASCVD including UA • Established clinical ASCVD plus diabetes or CKD greater than or equal to symbol three or HeFH • History of premature ASCVD (males: < 55; females: < 65)	LDL-C < 55; Non-HDL-C < 80; ApoB < 70; TG < 150
Very High	• Established or recent hospitalization (for ACS; carotid or peripheral vascular disease) or 10-year risk > 20% • Diabetes with 1+ risk factor • CKD greater than or equal to symbol three with albuminuria • HeFH	LDL-C < 70; Non-HDL-C < 100; ApoB < 80; TG < 150
High	• ≥ 2 risk factor & 10-year risk = 10 to 20% • Diabetes or CKD (≥ Stage 3) with no other risk factors	LDL-C < 100; Non-HDL-C < 130; ApoB < 90; TG < 150
Moderate	• < 2 risk factors & 10-year risk < 10%	LDL-C < 100; Non-HDL-C < 130; ApoB < 90; TG < 150
Low	• No risk factors	LDL-C < 130; Non-HDL-C < 160; ApoB = NR; TG < 150

Notes: AACE = American Association of Clinical Endocrinologists; UA = unstable angina; LDL-C = low-density lipoprotein cholesterol; HDL-C = high-density lipoprotein cholesterol; DM = diabetes mellitus; CKD = chronic kidney disease; HeFH = familial hypercholesterolemia; ACS = acute coronary syndrome; PVD = peripheral vascular disease; NR = not recommended.

Reference: Modified from Table 4 – AACE/ACE Management of Dyslipidemia and Prevention of Cardiovsacular Disease Algorithm Copyright © 2020 AACE.

Prepared by Erica Maceira and Jeanine Abrons; updated by Jeanine Abrons

Treating LDL-C to Goal in Patients with Diabetes

Risk Category	First Step	Based on LDL-C	
Extreme Risk	Lifestyle + high intensity statin	If LDL-C > 55 mg/dL: If LDL-C < 55 mg/dL:	• Step 2: Add PCKS9i, ezetimibe, colesevelam or bempedoic acid based on required LDL-C lowering • Step 3: Continue to add if not below desired LDL-C value
Very High Risk	Lifestyle + high intensity statin	If LDL-C > 70 mg/dL:	
High to Moderate Risk	Lifestyle + moderate intensity statin	If LDL-C > 100 mg/dL	• Step 2: Increase to high-intensity statin • Step 3: Add ezetimibe, colesevelam, or bempedoic acid • Step 4: Add agents to reach goal, consider PCSK9i
Low Risk	Lifestyle	If LDL-C > 130 mg/dL	• Step 2: Add moderate intensity statin • Step 3: Increase to high intensity statin • Step 4: Add ezetimibe, colesevelam, or bempedoic acid

*Note: Check lipids every three months or more frequently when necessary.

Statin Intensity-Based ASCVD Risk in Patients with Diabetes

Age	Patient with No Known Risk Factors	Patient with ASCVD Risk Factor(s)* or ASCVD Risk %	Patient has ASCVD
All ages	10-year	> 20%: high-intensity statin	High-intensity statin**
< 40	No statin therapy	Moderate or high-intensity statin*	High-intensity statin**
40 to 75	Moderate-intensity statin*	High-intensity statin	High-intensity statin**
> 75[a]	Moderate-intensity statin	Moderate or high-intensity statin	High-intensity statin**

a: If patient has change to acute coronary syndrome (ACS) and LDL cholesterol > 50 mg/dL and cannot tolerate high-dose statins, consider moderate-intensity statin dosing plus the addition of ezetimibe. For patients who do not tolerate the intended intensity, the maximally tolerated statin dose should be used. * = in addition to lifestyle therapy

**ASCVD risk factors include low-density lipoprotein (LDL) ≥ 100 mg/dL, high blood pressure, smoking, overweight or obesity, and family history of premature ASCVD; ***if LDL cholesterol ≥70 mg/dL despite maximally tolerated statin dose, consider adding other LDL-lowering therapy (such as ezetimibe or PCSK9 inhibitor)

Notes:
- If a patient is not taking a statin, it is reasonable to obtain a lipid profile at diabetes diagnosis, or at an initial medical evaluation, or every 5 years, or more often if indicated. Refer to ASCVD risk card for further guidance on initiating statin therapy.
- Recommendations for statin therapy should be made in addition to lifestyle therapy.
- Consider the following patients with diabetes mellitus (DM) to have similar risk to those with known CVD: men > age 40 with Type 2 + other coronary heart disease (CHD) risk factors OR age 50 with/without other CHD risk factors; women > 50 with Type 2 DM + other CHD risk factors OR age 55 with/without other CHD risk factors; men or women any age who have had DM for > 20 years with another risk factor OR men or women any age who have had DM > 25 years without another risk factor.

Reference: American Diabetes Association. Cardiovascular Disease and Risk Management: Standards of Medical Care in Diabetes—2021. Diabetes Care 2021 Jan; 44(Supplement 1):S125–S150.

Prepared by Jeanine P. Abrons, Molly Henry, and Elisha Andreas

Moderate and High-Intensity Statin Therapy

Moderate-Intensity Statins	High-Intensity Statins
Atorvastatin 10 to 20 mg; Rosuvastatin 5 to 10 mg; Simvastatin 20 to 40 mg; Pravastatin 40 to 80 mg; Lovastatin 40mg; Fluvastatin XL 80 mg; Pitavastatin 1 to 4 mg Expected LDL reduction = 30 to 49%	Atorvastatin 40 to 80 mg; Rosuvastatin 20 to 40 mg Expected LDL reduction = ≥ 50%

Updated by Emma Piehl and Jeanine Abrons.

Cholesterol Management:
Use of Drug Classes Other than Statins

Results other than high LDL-C
Some patients with metabolic syndrome also may have low HDL-C or high triglycerides. The AHA/ACC guidelines for prevention of coronary artery disease recommend consideration of additional medications directed at these lipids such as niacin and fibrates.

When to consider use of non-statins
May consider treatment with non-statin medications in high-risk patients with the following clinical scenarios:
- Less than anticipated response to statins (after compliance has been confirmed)
- Inability to tolerate a less than recommended intensity of statin
- Complete intolerance to statin therapy
- Fibrates & omega-3 fatty acids may be considered in patients with persistent triglycerides > 500 mg/dL after lifestyle modifications & treatment of causes
- Complete intolerance to statin therapy
- Consider PCSK9 (-) as an adjunct to maximally tolerated statin therapy for treatment of HeFH or clinical ASCVD who needed greater ↓ of LDL-cholesterol

High-risk patients include:
- Patients with clinical ASCVD
- Primary elevations of LDL-C > 190 mg/dL
- Patients with diabetes

Notes: LDL-C = low-density lipoprotein cholesterol; HDL-C = high-density lipoprotein cholesterol; PCSK9 = proprotein convertase subtilsin/kexin type 9; HeFH = heterozygous familial hypercholesterolemia; ASCVD = atherosclerotic cardiovascular disease.

Cholesterol Management:
Use of Drug Classes Other than Statins *(continued)*

Drug Classes Other Than Statins

Drug Class	Safety Considerations	Monitoring/Notes
Bile Acid Sequestrants	**Do not use if** • Fasting triglycerides (TG) > 300 mg/dL • Type III hyperlipoproteinemia **Use cautiously in patients with** • Triglycerides = 250 to 299 mg/dL **Discontinue use if** • TG increase to > 400 mg/dL	• Baseline: Fasting lipid profile • Re-evaluate 3 months after initiation and every 6 to 12 months thereafter
Cholesterol-Absorption Inhibitors (ezetimibe)	Discontinue with ALT (alanine aminotransferase) persistently > 3 times the upper limit of normal (ULN)	• Baseline: ALT/AST (aspartate transaminase) • When taken concomitantly with statins, monitor as clinically indicated • Monitor for CK ↑ associated with myopathy • May add with < 50% LDL-C ↓ while on high intensity statin • If TG > 300 mg/dL with use with statin, may add bile acid sequestrant
Fibrates	Gemfibrozil should not be used in conjunction with statins due to ↑ risk of muscle toxicities Fenofibrate may be considered in conjunction with low or moderate-intensity statins	• Renal function should be evaluated prior to initiation of fibrate, within 3 months of initiation, & every 6 months • Do not initiate, & discontinue if estimated glomerular filtration rate (eGFR) is persistently < 30 mL/min/1.73 m^2 • If eGFR is 30 to 59 mL/min/1.73 m^2, dose of fenofibrate should not be higher than 54 mg • Limited LDL lowering action & randomized controlled trials (RCTs) do not support use in addition to statins
Niacin	**Do not use if or with** • ALT/AST ≥ 2 to 3 times ULN • Persistent, severe cutaneous reactions occur • Hyperglycemia • Acute gout • Gastrointestinal (GI) symptoms • New onset atrial fibrillation OR • Weight loss occurs **When to use** • May consider niacin as adjunct for ↓ TG. Not for use with high-dose statins & well-controlled LDL cholesterol	• Baseline: ALT/AST, fasting blood glucose or A1c, uric acid • Re-evaluate during titration & every 6 months once maintenance dose is determined • Limited LDL lowering action & randomized controlled trials (RCTs) do not support use in addition to statins • In patients who develop cutaneous reactions: refer to guidelines • Re-evaluate use in patients who develop other side effects
Omega-3 Fatty Acids	• Minimal safety considerations	• Evaluate for GI disturbances, skin changes, & bleeding • Assess TG prior to initiating • Monitor for ↑ in bleeding time
PCSK9 Inhibitors	• Common ADRs include injection site reactions, URIs, & nasopharyngitis • Require subcutaneous administration	• Baseline: Fasting lipid panel • LDL-C: within 4 to 8 weeks of initiation or dose titration • Consider use in patients with very high risk & LDL-C ≥ 70 with statin therapy at max tolerated dose. ○ Use reasonable, but safety > 3 years is unknown/cost effectiveness if low.

Notes: CK = creatinine kinase; LDL = low-density lipoprotein; LDL-C = low-density lipoprotein cholesterol; ADR = adverse drug reaction; URI = upper respiratory infection.

Prepared by Nichole Bucci, Erica Maceira, Jeanine Abrons

Direct Oral Anticoagulants

Dabigatran (Pradaxa®)

Medication/Class/Notes on Use	Dabigatran (Pradaxa®) *Direct Thrombin Inhibitor (DTI)*
Indications T = Treatment P = Prophylaxis	• Stroke/emboli prevention in nonvalvular atrial fibrillation (NVAF)[T] • Deep vein thrombosis (DVT)/pulmonary embolism (PE) after 5 to 10 days of parenteral therapy[T] • ↓ DVT & PE recurrence in patients previously treated[P] • For DVT & PE prophylaxis in patients who have undergone hip & knee replacement
Usual Dosage T = Treatment P = Prophylaxis	<table><tr><th>Indication</th><th>T/P</th><th>Dose (Oral) = CrCl > 30mL/minute *After 5 to 10 days of parenteral therapy</th></tr><tr><td>NVAF</td><td>T</td><td>• 150 mg BID</td></tr><tr><td>DVT/PE*</td><td>T/P</td><td>• 150 mg BID • 150 mg BID after prior T</td></tr><tr><td>DVT/PE after hip replaced</td><td>P</td><td>• 110 mg on day 1, then 220 mg daily; start 1 to 4 hours after surgery/hemostasis achieved; for 28 to 35 days</td></tr></table>
Administration	• Must administer capsule whole with full glass of water; do not break, chew, crush, or open • Cannot administer per tube
Dose Adjustments *Based on Creatine Clearance (CrCl) using actual body weight*	<table><tr><th>Indication</th><th>T/P</th><th>Dose (Oral) = CrCl < 30mL/minute *After 5 to 10 days of parenteral therapy</th></tr><tr><td>NVAF</td><td>T</td><td>• CrCl 15 to 30 mL/min: 75 mg BID • CrCL < 15 mL/min or dialysis; not recommended</td></tr><tr><td>DVT/PE*</td><td>T</td><td>• At ≤ 30 mL/min: avoid use</td></tr><tr><td>DVT/PE after hip replaced</td><td>P</td><td>• At CrCl ≤ 30 mL/min or on dialysis: Dosing recommendations cannot be provided</td></tr></table>
Reversal	• Life threatening/uncontrolled bleeding/emergent surgery/urgent procedure: Idarucizumab (Praxbind®) 5 g IV single dose
Significant Drug Interactions	• Serious interactions & dose adjustments required with P-gp inducers/inhibitors, ketoconazole, & dronedarone – See PI for complete list
Miscellaneous Considerations	• Not recommended in end-stage renal disease (ESRD) • Do not use in antiphospholipid syndrome

CAD = coronary artery disease; PAD = peripheral artery disease; PI = package insert; DOC = drug of choice; TTR = time in therapeutic range for INR

Direct Oral Anticoagulants *(continued)*

Rivaroxaban (Xarelto®)

Medication/Class/Notes on Use	Rivaroxaban (Xarelto®) *Anti-Factor Xa Inhibitor*
Indications *T = Treatment* *P = Prophylaxis*	• Stoke/emboli prevention in NVAF[T] • DVT & PE[T] • DVT/PE risk ↓ after 6 months of prior treatment[P] • DVT/PE prophylaxis post hip/knee replacement • ↓ risk of cardiovascular events in CAD & PAD

Usual Dosage *T = Treatment* *P = Prophylaxis*	Indication	T/P	Dose (Oral)
	NVAF	T	• 20 mg daily
	DVT/PE	T	• 15 mg BID x 21 days, then 20 mg daily
		P	• After 6 months of therapy: 10 mg daily per PI after prior; take with food if patient does not need full anticoagulation
	Post Hip/ Knee Prophylaxis	P	• Knee: 10 mg daily x 12 days; start 6 to 10 hours post surgery • Hip: 10 mg daily x 35 days; start 6 to 10 hours post surgery
	Stable Coronary Artery Disease	P	• 2.5 mg BID in combo with Aspirin 75 to 100 mg daily
	Venous Thromboembolism in Acutely Ill Patients	P	• 10 mg daily for 35 days if started within 72 hours of hospitalization OR • 10 mg daily for 31 to 39 days (including hospitalization and post-discharge); extended prophylaxis should be avoided in patients with high risk of bleed
	Peripheral Artery Disease	P	• 2.5 mg BID in combo with Aspirin 75 to 100 mg daily

Administration	• Doses > 10 mg MUST be taken with food; best with **evening meal if dosed once daily for NVAF** test evening meal if dosed once daily for NVAF • Missed dosing based on frequency of dosing per day: For twice-daily treatment dosing, 2 doses may be taken at the same time to make up for missed dose • Can be crushed

Dose Adjustments *Based on Creatine Clearance* *(CrCl) Using Actual Body Weight*	Indication	T/P	Dose (Oral)
	NVAF	T	• CrCl 15 to 50 mL/min: 15 mg daily • CrCl < 15 mL/min: avoid use
	Post-Hip/ Knee Prophylaxis	T	• CrCl < 30 mL/min: avoid use
		P	• CrCl 30 to 50 mL/min: monitor for bleeding • Start 6 to 10 hours after surgery if adequate
	CV Risk ↓	P	• No adjustments needed based on CrCl

Reversal	• Life threatening/uncontrolled bleeding: Coagulation factor Xa (recombinant), inactivated-zhzo (Andexxa®) – Dosing based on specific Factor Xa Inhibitor (FXa), FXa dose, & time of last administration • Not dialyzable
Significant Drug Interactions	• Serious interactions & dose adjustments required with P-gp inducers/inhibitors, cytochrome P450 3A4 inducers/inhibitors – See PI
Miscellaneous Considerations	• Specifics of how to take is indication and dose specific • Not recommended in ESRD • Do not use in antiphospholipid syndrome

CAD = coronary artery disease; ESRD = end-stage renal disease; PAD = peripheral artery disease; PI = package insert;
DOC = drug of choice; TTR = time in therapeutic range for INR

Direct Oral Anticoagulants *(continued)*

Apixaban (Eliquis®)

Medication/Class/Notes on Use	Apixaban (Eliquis®) *Anti-factor Xa Inhibitor*
Indications *T = Treatment* *P = Prophylaxis*	• Stroke/emboli prevention in nonvalvular atrial fibrillation (NVAF)[T] • Deep vein thrombosis (DVT)/pulmonary embolism (PE)[T] • ↓ DVT & PE risk after prior T • DVT & PE prophylaxis in patients who have undergone hip & knee replacement[P]
Usual Dosage *T = Treatment* *P = Prophylaxis*	<table><tr><th>Indication</th><th>T/P</th><th>Dose (Oral) = CrCl > 30mL/minute</th></tr><tr><td>NVAF</td><td>T</td><td>• 5 mg BID</td></tr><tr><td rowspan="2">DVT Treatment</td><td>T</td><td>• 10 mg BID for 7 days, then 5 mg BID</td></tr><tr><td>P</td><td>• 2.5 mg BID after ≥ 6 months of T for DVT or PE</td></tr><tr><td>Post-Hip/ Knee Prophylaxis</td><td>P</td><td>• For Knee Replacement: 2.5 mg BID for 12 days; start 12 to 24 hours post surgery • For Hip Replacement: 2.5 mg BID for 35 days; start 12 to 24 hours post surgery</td></tr></table>
Administration	• Can be taken with or without food & can be crushed
Dose Adjustments ^ = *In dialysis may use dosing; Limited data to support use* *Based on Creatine Clearance (CrCl) Using Actual Body Weight*	<table><tr><th>Indication</th><th>T/P</th><th>Dose (Oral) = CrCl < 30mL/minute *After 5 to 10 days of parenteral therapy</th></tr><tr><td>NVAF</td><td>T</td><td>• If patient has any 2 traits: age ≥ 80, weight ≤ 60 kg, SCr ≥ 1.5 mg/dL: THEN 2.5 mg BID • CrCl < 15 mL/min not studied</td></tr><tr><td>DVT/PE Post-Knee/ Hip Prophylaxis</td><td>P</td><td>No dose adjustment for renal impairment for ESRD on dialysis; Use in CrCl < 15 mL/min not studied</td></tr></table>
Reversal	• Life threatening/uncontrolled bleeding: Coagulation factor Xa (recombinant), inactivated-zhzo (Andexxa®) – Dosing based on specific Factor Xa Inhibitor (FXa), FXa dose, & time of last administration
Significant Drug Interactions	• Serious interactions & dose adjustments required with dual use of P-gp inducers/ inhibitors, dual use of cytochrome P450 3A4 inducers/inhibitors – See PI for complete list
Miscellaneous Considerations	• Do not use in antiphospholipid syndrome

SCr = serum creatinine; PI = package insert; AHA = American Heart Association; ACC = American College of Cardiology

Direct Oral Anticoagulants *(continued)*

Edoxaban (Savaysa®)

Medication/Class/Notes on Use	Edoxaban (Savaysa®) *Anti-Factor Xa Inhibitor*
Indications T = Treatment P = Prophylaxis	• Stoke/emboli prevention in NVAF[T] • DVT/PE treatment after 5 to 10 days of parenteral anticoagulant[T]
Usual Dosage T = Treatment P = Prophylaxis	<table><tr><th>Indication</th><th>T/P</th><th>Dose (Oral) *After 5 to 10 days of parenteral therapy</th></tr><tr><td>NVAF</td><td>T</td><td>• 60 mg daily</td></tr><tr><td>DVT/PE</td><td>T P</td><td>• > 60 kg: 60 mg daily* • Less than or equal to 60 kg: 30 mg daily</td></tr></table>
Administration	• Can be taken with or without food • No data on crushing &/or mixing/giving through feeding tubes
Dose Adjustments ^ = In dialysis may use dosing; Limited data to support use *Based on Creatine Clearance (CrCl)*	<table><tr><th>Indication</th><th>T/P</th><th>Dose (Oral)</th></tr><tr><td>NVAF</td><td>T</td><td>• **Contraindicated in CrCl > 95 mL/min due to ↑ risk of ischemic stroke compared to warfarin** • At CrCl 15 to 50 mL/min: 15 mg daily • CrCl < 15 mL/minute: Not recommended • Patient weight ≤ 60 kg or with P-gp inhibitors or with short-term use of macrolide antibiotics: 30 mg daily</td></tr><tr><td>DVT/PE*</td><td>T</td><td>• At 15 to 50 mL/min or ≤ 60 kg who use certain P-gp inhibitors: 30 mg daily* • CrCl < 15 mL/minute: Not recommended</td></tr></table>
Reversal	• Hemodynamic support, PCC, and activated PCC may be considered
Significant Drug Interactions	Serious interactions & dose adjustments required with P-gp inhibitor in T of NVAF, for DVT/PE, ENGAGE-AF-TIMI 48: dose ↓ to ↓ levels compared to full dose T; DVT/PE: no dose ↓ with concomitant use – See PI for complete list
Miscellaneous Considerations	• Not recommended in ESRD • Do not use in antiphospholipid syndrome

NVAF = non-valvular atrial fibrillation; DVT = deep vein thrombosis; PE = pulmonary embolism; ESRD = end-stage renal disease; PCC = prothrombin complex concentrate

Prepared by: Erica Maceira, Nicole Bucci, and Shawn Phillips

Transitioning from Injectable Anticoagulants to Direct-Acting Oral Anticoagulants (DOACs)

Direct-Acting Oral Anticoagulant (DOAC)

Transition Being Pursued	Dabigatran Dose Transition Instructions	Apixaban Dose Transition Instructions
General Notes	• Initiate dabigatran within 2 hours prior to the time of the next scheduled dose of the parenteral anticoagulant.	• Initiate apixaban within 2 hours prior to the time of the next scheduled dose of the parenteral anticoagulant.
Transitioning from parenteral infusion	• Start dabigatran when infusion is stopped. • Consult local protocol if aPTT is above or below the target range.	• Start apixaban when the infusion is stopped. • Consult local protocol if the aPTT is above the target range.
Transitioning from warfarin	• Discontinue warfarin & initiate dabigatran when the INR is < 2.	• Discontinue warfarin and initiate apixaban as when the INR is < 2.
Transitioning to injectable anticoagulant/infusion	• After the last dose of dabigatran, wait 12 hours (CrCl ≥ 30 mL/min) or 24 hours (CrCl < 30 mL/min) before starting a parenteral anticoagulant.	• Start a parenteral anticoagulant when the next dose of apixaban is due.

Transitioning to warfarin	• Two options:
	1. Start warfarin the same day, & bridge with a parenteral anticoagulant until at INR goal.
	2. Overlap the two agents; the timing of warfarin initiation is based on CrCl:
	  ○ CrCl > 50 mL/min:
	   Initiate warfarin 3 days before discontinuing dabigatran.
	  ○ CrCl 30 to 50 mL/min:
	   Initiate warfarin 2 days before discontinuing dabigatran.
	  ○ CrCl 15 to 30 mL/min:
	   Initiate warfarin 1 day before discontinuing dabigatran.
		• Two options:
		1. Stop apixaban, start warfarin the same day. Bridge with a parenteral anticoagulant until a desired INR is reached.
		2. Bridge to warfarin with apixaban. To minimize interference, check INR near the end of apixaban dosing interval due to its impact on INR. Some experts suggest an overlap of apixaban with warfarin for ≥ 2 days until INR is therapeutic.

Transitioning to another DOAC	• Start the new DOAC when the next dose of the previous DOAC was scheduled to be given.	

*CrCl = Creatinine Clearance

Transitioning from Injectable Anticoagulants to Direct-Acting Oral Anticoagulants (DOACs) *(continued)*

Transition Being Pursued	Direct-Acting Oral Anticoagulant (DOAC)	
	Rivaroxaban	**Edoxaban**
General Notes	• Initiate rivaroxaban within 2 hours prior to the time of next scheduled dose of the parenteral anticoagulant.	• Initiate edoxaban within 2 hours prior to the time of the next scheduled dose of the parenteral anticoagulant.
Transitioning from parenteral infusion	• Start rivaroxaban when the infusion is stopped (consult local protocol if aPTT is above the target range).	• N/A
Transitioning from warfarin	• Discontinue warfarin & start rivaroxaban as soon as INR falls to <3.	• Discontinue warfarin & initiate edoxaban as soon as INR falls to ≤2.5.
Transitioning from LMWH or Fondaparinux	• Start rivaroxaban prior to the next scheduled dose of the parenteral agent.	• N/A
Transitioning to injectable anticoagulant/infusion	• Start the parenteral anticoagulant when the next dose of rivaroxaban was scheduled to be given.	• Start the parenteral anticoagulant when the next dose of edoxaban was scheduled to be given.
Transitioning to warfarin	Two options: 1. Stop rivaroxaban, start warfarin the same day, & bridge with a parenteral anticoagulant until the desired INR is reached. 2. Bridge to warfarin with rivaroxaban. To minimize interference, check INR near the end of rivaroxaban's dosing interval due to INR impact. Some experts suggest overlapping apixaban with warfarin for ≥ 2 days until INR is therapeutic. 3. Start rivaroxaban when the infusion is stopped (consult local protocol if aPTT is above the target range).	Two options: 1. For patients taking edoxaban 60 mg once daily, ↓ the dose to 30 mg once daily & begin warfarin. For patients taking edoxaban 30 mg once daily, ↓ the dose to 15 mg once daily & begin warfarin. Monitor INR at the end of edoxaban dosing due to INR impact. Discontinue edoxaban once INR is stable at ≥ 2. 2. Stop edoxaban, start warfarin the same day, & bridge with a parenteral anticoagulant until the desired INR is reached.
Transitioning from parenteral Infusion		• N/A
Transitioning to another DOAC	• Start the new DOAC when the next dose of the previous DOAC was scheduled to be given.	

*CrCl = Creatinine Clearance; N/A = not applicable

Injectable Anticoagulants

Injectable Anticoagulant/ Consideration	Unfractionated Heparin	Enoxaparin (Lovenox®)	Dalteparin (Fragmin®)	Fondaparinux (Arixtra®)
Dosing				
Prophylaxis	• 5000 units SC every 8 hours or 5000 units SC every 12 hours	• 30 mg SC every 12 hours OR 40 mg SC every 24 hours • Creatinine clearance (CrCl) < 30 mL/min: 30 mg SC every 24 hours • Use in dialysis has limited data (not dialyzable)	• 5000 units SC every 24 hours • Postsurgical prophylaxis for abdominal surgery: 2500 units SC every 24 hours • Postsurgical prophylaxis hip replacement: 2500 units 2 hours prior to surgery, then 2500 units 4 hours (or longer if failure to achieve hemostasis) after surgery, then 5000 units SC every 24 hours • Do not use in dialysis	• 2.5 mg SC every 24 hours • Do not use in patients with CrCl < 30 mL/min or patients < 50 kg
VTE Treatment	• SC: 333 units/kg SC once followed by 250 units/kg SC every 12 hours • IV: 80 units/kg or 5000 units IV bolus, then infusion of 18 units/kg (or 1000 units/hour) titrated to APTT or antifactor Xa assay (anti-Xa) • Goal: APTT = 1.5 to 2.5 x normal, anti-Xa = 0.3 to 0.7	• 1 mg/kg SC every 12 hours OR • 1.5 mg/kg SC every 24 hours • CrCl < 30 mL/min: 1 mg/kg SC every 24 hours • Do not use in dialysis	• 100 units/kg SC every 12 hours OR • 200 units SC every 24 hours • Do not use in patients with CrCl < 30 mL/min	• < 50 kg: 5 mg SC every 24 hours • 50 to 100 kg: 7.5 mg SC every 24 hours • > 100 kg: 10 mg SC every 24 hours • Do not use in patients with CrCl < 30 mL/min
Half-life	• 1 to 2 hours • Impacted by obesity; renal function; malignancy; & presence of pulmonary embolism	• 5 to 7 hours • Impacted by renal function, pregnancy, obesity, & cumulative dose	• 2 to 5 hours • Impacted by renal function	• 17 to 21 hours • Impacted by renal function
Excretion	• Primarily hepatic but also by reticuloendothelial system • Higher dose: renal elimination may play more of a role	• Excretion: impacted by renal function, pregnancy, obesity, & cumulative dose	• Excretion: primarily renal (dose dependent)	• Excretion: urine (77% excreted unchanged)
Inhibited Factors	• Factors IIa, IXa, Xa, XIa, XIIa • Plasmin	• Factors Xa & IIa	• Factors Xa & IIa	• Factor Xa

Notes: All act through antithrombin III (so in patients with antithrombin III deficiency, these agents will predominantly be ineffective depending on the degree of deficiency). SC = subcutaneous; IV = intravenous; VTE = venous thromboembolism; APTT = activated partial thromboplastin time.

Prepared by: Erica Maceira, Nicole Bucci, and Shawn Phillips

Injectable Anticoagulants *(continued)*

Direct Thrombin Inhibitors (DTIs)

Injectable Anticoagulant/ Consideration	Argatroban	Bivalrudin (Angiomax®)
Indications	• Prophylaxis of coronary artery thrombosis in percutaneous coronary intervention patients with or at risk for HIT* • HIT treatment & prophylaxis*	• Anticoagulant use for patients undergoing PCI* • Management of HIT** • Off-label dosing also listed for ischemic heart and NSTEMI

Usual Dose	• Prophylaxis in PCI:[ƒ]
	  ○ 350 mcg/kg bolus over 3 min, then 35 mcg/kg/min IV continuous infusion
	  ○ Can re-bolus at 150 mcg/kg &/or ↑ rate to a maximum of 40 mcg/kg/min to achieve clotting time of 300 to 450 seconds
	• HIT treatment & prophylaxis:
	  ○ 2 mcg/kg/min continuous IV infusion; adjust until APTT is 1.5 to 3 times baseline to a maximum of 10 mcg/kg/min
		• During PCI for ACS:
		  ○ 0.75 mg/kg/bolus prior to procedure, followed by 1.75 mg/kg/hour for procedure duration; extended duration of infusion (up to 4 hours). Monitor ACT 5 min after bolus; give additional bolus of 0.3 mg/kg if needed.
		  ○ Bolus & infusion different if initiating prior to PCI.
		• Off-label dosing for HIT:
		  ○ Data suggests dosing of 0.15 mg/kg/hour titrated to APTT 1.5 to 3 times control
		• Cardiac surgery in patients with acute/subacute HIT:
		  ○ Off-pump/on-pump dosing available

Dose Adjustments	• HIT treatment & prophylaxis with severe hepatic disease:
	  ○ Start at a rate of 0.5 mcg/kg/min
		• During PCI:
		  ○ No ↓ in bolus dose required for any degree of renal impairment
		  ○ CrCl < 30 mL/min: ↓ infusion rate to 1 mg/kg/hour
		  ○ ESRD on HD: ↓ infusion rate to 0.25 mg/kg/hour
		• Off-label dosing for HIT:
		  ○ CrCl = 30 to 59 mL/min: 0.08 mg/kg/hour
		  ○ CrCl < 30 mL/min: 0.03 mg/kg/hour
		• Dialyzable: May require dose adjustments

Onset	• Immediate	• Immediate
Half-life	• 30 min to 1 hour • ↑ in severe hepatic impairment to as high as 3 hours	• 25 min to 3.5 hours • Impacted by renal function
Excretion	• 25% renal; 16% unchanged • 65% fecal; 14% unchanged	• Excretion: Renal (dose dependent)
Inhibited Factors	• Factor II	• Factor II
Lab Interference	• When given with warfarin during bridging can falsely elevate INR due to lab interference • Lab interference (impact on INR) is dose related—higher doses have greater impact on INR (some institutions & PI recommend decrease of infusion rate down to 2/kg)	• PT/INR levels may ↑ in the absence of warfarin. If warfarin initiated, consider modification of initial PT/INR goals. • May need to consider modification of therapy depending on impact

Notes: * = FDA-approved indication; ** = off-label use; ƒ = multiple possible doses for this indication. HIT = heparin-induced thrombocytopenia; SC = subcutaneous; IV = intravenous; PCI = percutaneous coronary intervention; ACS = acute coronary syndrome; ACT = activated clotting time; CrCl = creatinine clearance; ESRD = end-stage renal disease; HD = hemodialysis; APTT = activated partial thromboplasty time; INR = international normalized ratio; PT = prothrombin time; NSTEMI = non-ST-elevation myocardial infarction.

Prepared by Erica Maceira, Shawn Phillips, Nicole Bucci

Perioperative Management of Direct Oral Anticoagulants

Medication/ Renal Function (Creatinine Clearance [CrCl])	Half Life (T ½)	Low Bleeding Risk Surgery: Timing of Last Dose	High Bleeding Risk Surgery: Timing of Last Dose	When to Resume Therapy — LOW Bleeding Risk Surgery	When to Resume Therapy — HIGH Bleeding Risk Surgery
Dabigatran (Pradaxa®)					
>50 mL/min	T ½ = 12 to 17 hours; 14 to 17 hours in elderly	2 days before procedure	3 days before procedure	Resume on the day after procedure (24 hours postoperative)	Resume 2 to 3 days after procedure (48 to 72 hours postoperative)
30 to 50 mL/min	T ½ = 15 to 18 hours	3 days before procedure	4 to 5 days before procedure		
Rivaroxaban (Xarelto®)					
>30 mL/min	T ½ = 5 to 9 hours	At least 1 day before procedure	At least 2 days before procedure	Resume on the day after procedure (24 hours postoperative)	Resume 2 to 3 days after procedure (48 to 72 hours postoperative)
<30 mL/min	T ½ = 9 to 10 hours	2 days before procedure	3 days before procedure		
Apixaban (Eliquis®)					
>30 mL/min	T ½ = 12 to 18 hours	1 day before procedure	2 days before procedure	Resume on the day after procedure (24 hours postoperative)	Resume 2 to 3 days after procedure (48 to 72 hours postoperative)
<30 mL/min	T ½ = ~17 hours	2 days before procedure	3 days before procedure		
Edoxaban (Savaysa®)					
>50 mL/min	T ½ = 10 to 14 hours	2 days before procedure	3 days before procedure	Resume on the day after procedure (24 hours postoperative)	Resume 2 to 3 days after procedure (48 to 72 hours postoperative)

Note: For patients at high risk for thromboembolism and bleed risk after surgery, consider administering a reduced dose of dabigatran (75 mg BID), rivaroxaban (10 mg daily), or apixaban (2.5 mg BID) on the evening after surgery and on the first postoperative day; bridging is not indicated with DOACs due to the predictable pharmacokinetics.

These recommendations are for patients not undergoing neuraxial procedures. For patients undergoing neuraxial procedures, see the American Society of Regional Anesthesia & Pain Medicine guidelines: https://journals.lww.com/rapm/Fulltext/2015/05000/Interventional_Spine_and_Pain_Procedures_in.2.aspx (Accessed 2021).

Reference: Doherty J, Gluckman T, Hucker W, et al. 2017 ACC Expert Consensus Decision Pathway for Periprocedural Management of Anticoagulation in Patients With Nonvalvular Atrial Fibrillation: A Report of the American College of Cardiology Clinical Expert Consensus Document Task Force. J Am Coll Cardiol. 2017 Feb 21;69(7):871–898.

Prepared by Erica Maceria and Apryl Jacobs

Common Warfarin Drug Interactions

Drug Class or Medication That Interacts with Warfarin	Impact on Warfarin levels: Potential Management
Antibiotics E.g., ciprofloxacin; clarithromycin; erythromycin; metronidazole; sulfamethoxazole/trimethoprim	Majority ↑
	Metronidazole: ↑; consider alternatives. If used together, consider ↓ warfarin dose by 25 to 50% — **Dicloxacillin:** ↓; more significant if course >14 days
	Rifampin: ↓; may consider ↑ of warfarin dose by 25 to 50%. — **Ciprofloxacin:** ↑ At 2 to 5 days; may consider ↓ warfarin dose by 10 to 15%
	Clarithromycin: At 3 to 7 days; may ↓ dose warfarin 15 to 25% — **Erythromycin:** At 3 to 5 days; may consider ↓ warfarin dose by 10 to 15%
	Sulfamethoxazole/Trimethoprim: ↑ At 2 to 5 days; may consider ↓ warfarin dose by 25 to 40%; consider alternative antibiotic due to severity of interaction
Antifungal Medications: E.g., fluconazole; miconazole	↑; At 2 to 3 days; consider initial dose ↓ by 25 to 30%; may need to ↓ up to 80% with fluconazole
Antidepressants: E.g., quetiapine; SSRIs	↑; **Trazodone:** Warfarin dose may need to be ↓ by 25 to 30%
Antiplatelet Medications	Does not increase INR, just ↑ bleeding risk. Monitor for signs/symptoms.
Anticoagulant Medications	Generally does not increase INR, just ↑ bleeding risk. Monitor for signs/symptoms. Argatroban & bivalirudin can ↑ INR; when bridging with these medications, this ↑ should be considered
Amiodarone	↑; slow ↑ over time (e.g., 6 to 8 weeks); empiric warfarin dose by 10 to 25% at week 1; may ↓ warfarin dose by 25 to 60% eventually
Acetaminophen	↑; with high doses (limited dose to < 2000 mg/day → avoid use of higher doses if possible); onset at 2 to 5 days
Carbamazepine	↓; warfarin dose may need to be ↑ by 50 to 100%; ↓ warfarin dose by 50% when stopping
Fenofibrate	↑; warfarin dose may need to be ↓ by 50 to 100%; ↑ warfarin dose by 50% when stopping
Gemfibrozil	↑; may ↓ dose warfarin by 10 to 15%
Phenobarbital	↓; warfarin dose may need to be ↑ by 30 to 60%
Phenytoin as drug or medication	Interaction with warfarin is biphasic—initially will ↑ the INR, typically first couple of months, then can ↓ INR. Warfarin can ↑ phenytoin levels—monitor levels
Rosuvastatin	↑; may ↓ dose warfarin by 10 to 25%
	↑ Levels — **↓ Levels**
Alternative Therapies Note: Please refer to additional reference for more extensive list	C: cannabis; capsicum; chamomile; clove; cranberry — G: ginseng; green tea; goldenseal
	G: garlic; ginger; gingko; grapefruit — Other: noni; parsley; St. John's wort; yarrow

Notes: For all significant drug interactions, monitor international normalized ratio (INR) more often.

This table is not all inclusive; it provides a guidance for recall of drug interactions that require dose adjustment of warfarin; e.g., anti-inflammatory & antiplatelet medications should have increased monitoring for signs & symptoms of bleeding; SSRI = selective serotonin reuptake inhibitor.

Sample References: http://www.ncbi.nlm.nih.gov/pmc/articles/PMC1942100/pdf/20070814s00019p369.pdf (Accessed 2021); Alternative Therapies Reference: National Center for Complementary and Alternative Medicine (http://nccam.nih.gov/health/herbsataglance.html (Accessed 2021).

Prepared by Jeanine P. Abrons and Erica Maceira

Warfarin Dosing Principles

Monitoring of Warfarin:
- In hospitalized patients, INR monitoring is often performed daily until therapeutic range is maintained for 2 consecutive days.
- In an outpatient setting, INRs are monitored more often initially (e.g., every 1 to 3 days), & then the frequency between INRs can be once a stable dose is achieved.
- For outpatients with stable INRs, the testing frequency may be extended up to 12 weeks (rather than every 4 weeks).
- The optimal frequency of monitoring may be impacted by patient compliance, comorbid considerations, medication use, adherence, warfarin sensitivity, presence of signs/symptoms of bleeding, & dose response.

Consider the influence of factors associated with increased warfarin sensitivity:

• Age > 65	• Heart failure
• Cirrhosis or total bilirubin > 2.4 g/dL	• Alcohol abuse history
• Hypoalbuminemia < 2 g/dL	• Surgery within 2 weeks
• End stage renal disease (ESRD)	• Chronic diarrhea
• Bleeding: GI bleed or intracranial bleed within 30 days	• Malnourished or nothing by mouth (NPO) for > 3 days
• Actual body weight (ABW) < 45 kg or ABW < ideal	• Thrombocytopenia: platelets < 75 k/uL
• Other medications: e.g., antiplatelet drugs, other drug interactions, etc.	

If fluctuations occur – consider the reason for the fluctuation:

• Inaccuracy of INR testing	• Changes in dietary vitamin K intake
• Changes in absorption, distribution, metabolism, & excretion of vitamin K or warfarin	• Concomitant medical conditions

Management of out-of-range INRs:
- For previously stable patients with a single out-of-range INR of ≤ 0.5 below or above the therapeutic range, the current dose may be continued & testing can be done within 1 to 2 weeks.
- With major bleeding, rapid reversal of anticoagulation with four-factor prothrombin complex concentrate is suggested rather than with plasma.
- Add vitamin K 5 to 10 mg oral or intravenous rather than reversal with coagulation factors alone.

Management of out-of-range INRs:

INR Level and Evidence of Bleeding	Recommendation
4.5 to 10 & No Evidence of Bleeding	Routine vitamin K use not recommended
> 10 & No Evidence of Bleeding	Administer oral vitamin K
Evidence of Bleeding	Kcentra® & vitamin K

Target INRs:
- Therapeutic INRs of 2 to 3 rather than lower (< 2) or higher (3 to 5) are recommended for most indications.
- Higher-intensity INR ranges exist for patients with mechanical mitral valves or with mechanical aortic valve & other risk factors.

Warfarin Dosing Principles *(continued)*

Initiation of warfarin dosing based on CHEST Guidelines:
- Sufficiently healthy patients to be treated as outpatients may start at 10 mg for 2 days followed by dosing based on INR.
- In patients with acute thromboembolism, therapy may be started on day 1 or 2 of an injectable anticoagulant rather than waiting to start.
- Many patients will be started at doses between 5 & 10 mg.
- A starting dose of < 5 mg may be considered in: elderly, impaired nutrition, liver disease, high bleeding risk, & congestive heart failure.
- 2 to 3 mg initial dose appropriate for patient with heart valve replacement.

Other points related to warfarin:
- Many drug interactions exist. Discuss the likelihood of a drug interaction & encourage patients to report all medication changes.
- In patients with recurrent venous thromboembolism (in therapeutic range & believed to be compliant), it is suggested to switch treatment to LMWH at least temporarily while further assessments are made.

Consistency is key with:

• Medication adherence/interactions	• INR monitoring
• For enteral nutrition: holding tube feed 1 hour before/after warfarin	• Vitamin K intake

Ask questions if recent changes have occurred:

• Does the new med interact?	• Has there been recent illness?
• Have there been dietary changes?	• How does patient take medication (assess adherence)?

Signs & symptoms of bleeding:
- Stress the importance of reporting signs or symptoms to the doctor & pharmacist.
- This may mean that warfarin is dosed at too high a level or that further monitoring is needed.

Warfarin Strengths and Colors

1 mg:	2 mg:	2.5 mg:	3 mg:	4 mg:	5 mg:	6 mg:	7.5 mg:	10 mg:
Pink	Purple	Green	Brown	Blue	Orange	Teal	Yellow	White

Other Warfarin Resources (Accessed 2021)

- http://www.warfarindosing.org
- http://www.coumadin.bmscustomerconnect.com
- Witt DM, Clark NP, Kaatz S, Schnurr T, Ansell JE. Guidance for the practical management of warfarin therapy in the treatment of venous thromboembolism. *Journal of thrombosis thrombolysis*. 2016 Jan 1;41(1):187–205.

Prepared by Jeanine P. Abrons

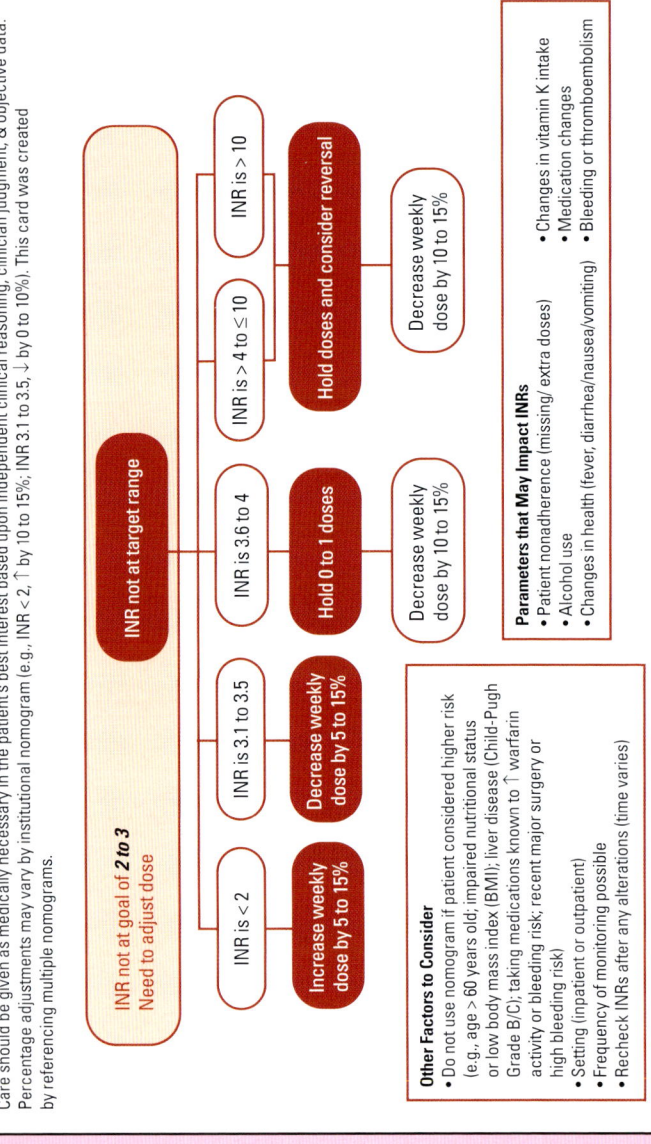

Alterations to Warfarin Dose Maintenance Therapy

This flowchart does not replace the need for clinical decision making. Decisions regarding patient care should be made in accordance with clinical judgment. Care should be given as medically necessary in the patient's best interest based upon independent clinical reasoning, clinician judgment, & objective data. Percentage adjustments may vary by institutional nomogram (e.g., INR < 2, ↑ by 10 to 15%; INR 3.1 to 3.5, ↓ by 0 to 10%). This card was created by referencing multiple nomograms.

INR not at goal of *2 to 3* — Need to adjust dose

INR not at target range

- **INR is < 2** → Increase weekly dose by 5 to 15%
- **INR is 3.1 to 3.5** → Decrease weekly dose by 5 to 15%
- **INR is 3.6 to 4** → Hold 0 to 1 doses → Decrease weekly dose by 10 to 15%
- **INR is > 4 to ≤ 10** → Hold doses and consider reversal → Decrease weekly dose by 10 to 15%
- **INR is > 10** → Hold doses and consider reversal → Decrease weekly dose by 10 to 15%

Other Factors to Consider
- Do not use nomogram if patient considered higher risk (e.g., age > 60 years old; impaired nutritional status or low body mass index [BMI]; liver disease (Child-Pugh Grade B/C); taking medications known to ↑ warfarin activity or bleeding risk; recent major surgery or high bleeding risk)
- Setting (inpatient or outpatient)
- Frequency of monitoring possible
- Recheck INRs after any alterations (time varies)

Parameters that May Impact INRs
- Patient nonadherence (missing/ extra doses)
- Alcohol use
- Changes in health (fever, diarrhea/nausea/vomiting)
- Changes in vitamin K intake
- Medication changes
- Bleeding or thromboembolism

APhA

Alterations to Warfarin Dose Maintenance Therapy *(continued)*

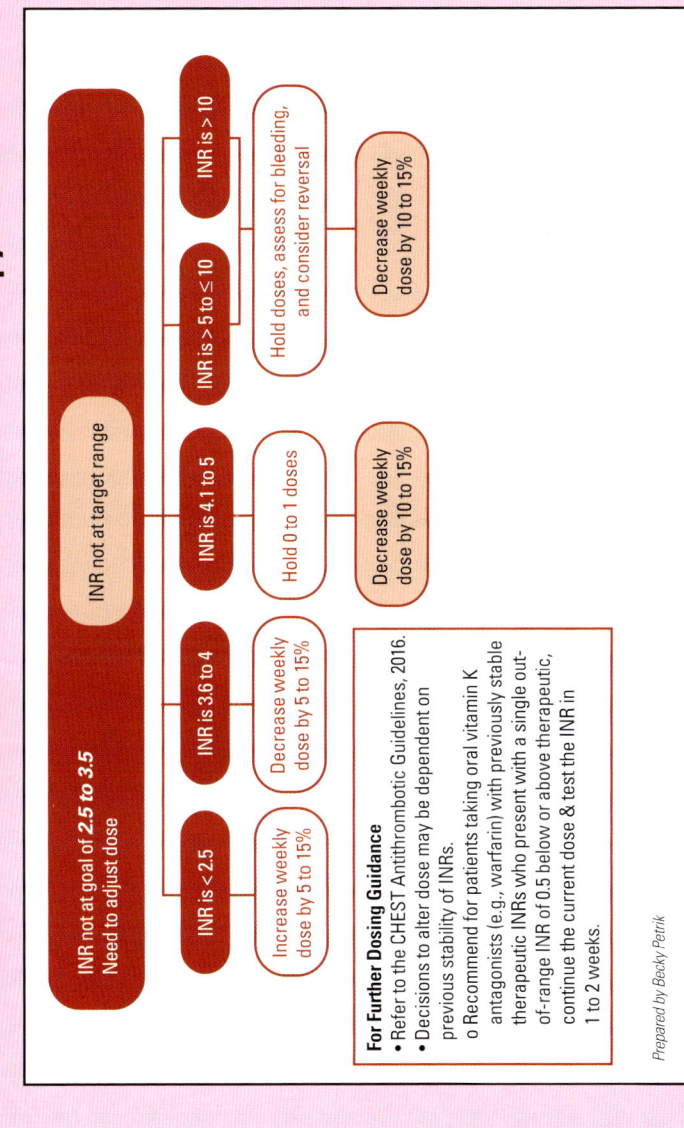

INR not at goal of 2.5 to 3.5 — Need to adjust dose

INR not at target range

- **INR is < 2.5** → Increase weekly dose by 5 to 15%
- **INR is 3.6 to 4** → Decrease weekly dose by 5 to 15%
- **INR is 4.1 to 5** → Hold 0 to 1 doses → Decrease weekly dose by 10 to 15%
- **INR is > 5 to ≤ 10** → Hold doses, assess for bleeding, and consider reversal → Decrease weekly dose by 10 to 15%
- **INR is > 10** → Hold doses, assess for bleeding, and consider reversal → Decrease weekly dose by 10 to 15%

For Further Dosing Guidance
- Refer to the CHEST Antithrombotic Guidelines, 2016.
- Decisions to alter dose may be dependent on previous stability of INRs.
  - Recommend for patients taking oral vitamin K antagonists (e.g., warfarin) with previously stable therapeutic INRs who present with a single out-of-range INR of 0.5 below or above therapeutic, continue the current dose & test the INR in 1 to 2 weeks.

Prepared by Becky Petrik

ACLS Drugs by Arrhythmia Type or Condition

Arrhythmia	Medication(s) Used
Ventricular Fibrillation (VF)	Amiodarone
	Epinephrine
	Lidocaine (if amiodarone unavailable)
	Magnesium (if QT prolongation)
Stable Ventricular Tachycardia (VT)	Adenosine
	Amiodarone
Pulseless Ventricular Tachycardia	Amiodarone
	Epinephrine
	Lidocaine (if amiodarone unavailable)
	Magnesium (if QT prolongation)
Stable Narrow-QRS VT	Adenosine
	Beta blocker/calcium channel blocker (i.e., diltiazem)
Stable Wide-QRS VT	Adenosine
	Procainamide
	Lidocaine
	Sotalol
Supraventricular Tachycardia	Diltiazem
	Procainamide
Paroxysmal Supraventricular Tachycardia (PSVT)	Adenosine
Monomorphic VT	Sotalol
Stable Polymorphic VT/Torsade's de Pointes	Magnesium (if QT prolongation)
Asystole/Pulseless Electrical Activity	Epinephrine
Bradycardia	Atropine
	Epinephrine
Shock/Hypotension	Epinephrine
	Norepinephrine
	Vasopressin

Note: Drugs are listed in alphabetic order that can be used for a given indication not as order of use. ACLS References: Lexicomp [database online]. Hudson, OH: Wolters Kluwer Clinical Drug Information, Inc. 2020. http://online.lex.com/. (Accessed November 2021); ACLS Cardiac Arrest, Arrhythmias and Their Treatment. 15–1007(1 of 2)ISBN 978-1-61669-402-9 3/16
© 2016 American Heart Association. Printed in the USA.

Diabetes Treatment Guidelines

For more comprehensive information about current approaches to the diagnosis and treatment of diabetes, visit the American Diabetes Association Standards of Medical Care—2022 website at *https://diabetesjournals.org/care/issue/45/Supplement_1* (Accessed 2022).

Criteria for Defining Prediabetes & Diagnosis of Diabetes

Diagnostic Tool	Prediabetes Criteria	Value Associated with Diagnosis of Diabetes
Fasting Plasma Glucose (FPG)[a]	100 to 125 mg/dL	$\geq$ 126 mg/dL • In absence of unequivocal hyperglycemia, diagnosis requires two abnormal test results from the same sample or two separate samples
Random Plasma Glucose	No recommendations	$\geq$ 200 mg/dL with symptoms (polyuria; polydipsia; unexplained weight loss) • Value measured without regard to last meal • Only diagnostic with classic symptoms of hyperglycemia or hyperglycemic crisis
Oral Glucose Tolerance Test	140 to 199 mg/dL	$\geq$ 200 mg/dL 2 hours post 75 g oral glucose tolerance test (OGTT) glucose challenge • In absence of unequivocal hyperglycemia, diagnosis requires two abnormal test results from the same sample or two separate samples
Hemoglobin A1c[b]	5.7 to 6.4%	$\geq$ 6.5% • Performed in a laboratory using a method that is NGSP certified[c] & standardized to the DCCT assay[d]

a: Definition of fasting: no caloric intake for at least 8 hours.

b: In conditions associated with ↑ red blood cell turnover (e.g., sickle cell disease, pregnancy [2nd & 3rd trimester], hemodialysis, recent blood loss/transfusion, or erythropoietin therapy): Only plasma blood glucose should be used to diagnose diabetes.

c: National Glycohemoglobin Standardization Program.

d: Diabetes Control & Complications Trial.

Practitioner may select one diagnostic tool above and in absence of unequivocal hyperglycemia should confirm results with repeat testing.

Note: Patients age 45 years old, with body mass index (BMI) > 25 kg/m² or > 23 kg/m² in Asian Americans, &/or adults with $\geq$ 1 risk factor, even if asymptomatic, should be screened for diabetes with the above diagnostic tools and criteria. Risk factors include first-degree relative with diabetes; high-risk race/ethnicity (e.g., African American, Latino, Native American, Asian American, Pacific Islander); history of cardiovascular disease; hypertension (> 140/90 mmHg or on therapy for hypertension); HDL < 35 mg/dL &/or a triglyceride level > 250 mg/dL; women with polycystic ovarian syndrome; physical inactivity; other clinical conditions associated with insulin resistance (e.g., severe obesity, acanthosis nigricans). For all patients, testing should be initiated at age 45 & offered at 3-year intervals with more frequent testing depending on initial results & risk status. In patients with prediabetes or increased risk for diabetes, testing should be done more frequently (yearly). Additional testing & screening information available with cystic fibrosis, posttransplantation, gestational diabetes, & monogenic diabetes syndromes.

Criteria for Testing for Diabetes or Pre-Diabetes in Asymptomatic Adults

Consider screening in:
- Overweight or obese (BMI $\geq$ 25 kg/m²) who have one or more risk factor:
  – First-degree relative with diabetes
  – High-risk race/ethnicity (e.g., African American, Latino, Native American, Pacific Islander, Asian American)
  – History of cardiovascular disease (CVD)
  – Hypertension ($\geq$ 140/90 mmHg or on therapy for hypertension)
  – High density lipoprotein (HDL) cholesterol level < 35 mg/dL &/or a triglyceride level > 250 mg/dL
  – Women with polycystic ovary syndrome
  – Physical inactivity
  – Other clinical conditions associated with insulin resistance (e.g., severe obesity, acanthosis nigricans)
  – HIV

Consider yearly screening in:
- Patients with pre-diabetes (A1c $\geq$ 5.7%)

Lifelong screening every 3 years:
- Women who were diagnosed with gestational diabetes

Screen after age 35:
- For all other patients, testing should begin at age 45 years
- If results are normal, testing should be repeated at a minimum of 3-year intervals; see guidelines for additional information if pre-diabetes is identified.

Updated by Emma Piehl, Jeanine P. Abrons, Elisha Andreas, and Molly Henry.

Patient-Centered Glycemic Collaborative Care in the Management in Type 2 Diabetes Decision Cycle

Area of Care	Description of Care
Assess key patient characteristics	• Current lifestyle • Comorbidities (e.g., ASCVD, CKD, Heart Failure) • Clinical characteristics (e.g., age, hemoglobin A1c, weight) • Issues such as motivation & depression • Cultural & socioeconomic context
Consider specific factors that impact the choice of treatment	• Individualized hemoglobin A1c target • Impact on weight & hypoglycemia • Side-effect profile of medication • Complexity of regimen (e.g., frequency, mode of administration) • A regimen that optimizes adherence & persistence • Access, cost, & availability of medication • Social life assessment (e.g., food insecurity, housing stability, financial & language barriers)
Create a management plan with shared decision making	• Involves an educated & informed patient or family caregiver • Seeks patient preferences • Empowers the patient • Effective consultation with motivational interviewing, goal setting, & shared decision making • Refer patients to local resources & ensure access to Diabetes Self-Management Education & Support (DSMES) by health coaches, community health workers, etc.
Agree on the management plan	• SMART goals (Specific; Measurable; Achievable; Realistic; Time-limited)
Implement the management plan	• Patients not meeting goals generally should be seen at least every 3 months if progress is being made; more frequent initial contact is desirable for DSMES
Provide ongoing monitoring and support	Provide monitoring and support to evaluate the following • Emotional well-being • Tolerability of medication • Glycemic status • Biofeedback (e.g., self-monitoring of blood glucose, weight, step count, hemoglobin A1c, blood pressure, & lipids)
Review and agree on a management plan	• Review management plan • Mutually agree on changes • Ensure the modification of therapy is implemented in a timely manner to avoid clinical inertia • Undertake a decision cycle regularly (at least once or twice a year)
Overall goals	Overall goals are to: • Prevent complications • Optimize quality of life

American Diabetes Association. Standards of Medical Care in Diabetes—2022. Diabetes: *https://diabetesjournals.org/care/issue/45/Supplement_1 (Accessed 2022)*

Prepared by Jeanine Abrons and Elisha Andreas; updated by Emma Piehl and Jeanine Abrons

Associated Goals for Adults with Diabetes

Associated Goals	Value of Goal
Glycemic Control (A1c)[a]	ADA*: Less stringent for patients at risk for severe hypoglycemiaor < 7%[b]
	AACE**: < 6.5%[c]
Preprandial Capillary Plasma Glucose	ADA: 80 to 130 mg/dL[b]
	AACE: < 110 mg/dL
Peak Postprandial Capillary Plasma Glucose	ADA: < 180 mg/dL[b,d]
	AACE: < 140 mg/dL
Blood Pressure	ADA: Patients with diabetes & hypertension at ↑ cardiovascular risk (existing ASCVD or 10-year ASCVD risk $\geq$ 15%): < 130/80 mmHg
	Patients with diabetes & hypertension at lower cardiovascular risk (10 year ASCVD risk <15%): < 140/90 mmHg
	In pregnant patients: < 110 to 135/85 mmHg
	AACE: < 130/80 mmHg[e]

Notes: *American Diabetes Association (ADA) Standards of Medical Care 2022; **American Association of Clinical Endocrinologists (AACE) & American College of Endocrinology Comprehensive Type 2 Diabetes Management Algorithm 2020.

a: Perform A1c testing at least 2 times per year in patients meeting treatment goals (and who have stable glycemic control). Perform A1c testing quarterly in patients with changes to therapy or who are not meeting glycemic goals.

b: More or less stringent glycemic goals may be appropriate for each patients. Less stringent may be considered in patients with increased risk of hypoglycemia, limited life expectancy, advanced microvascular or macrovascular complications, extensive co-morbid conditions, or long-standing diabetes when goals are difficult to achieve despite self-management education, appropriate monitoring, & effective dosing of therapies, patient preference & limits to resources/support system. More stringent may be considered for patients with short duration of diabetes, type 2 diabetes treated with lifestyle interventions or metformin only, long-life expectancy, or no significant cardiovascular disease.

c: For patients without concurrent serious illness & at low hypoglycemic risk; level $\geq$ 6.5% for patients with concurrent illness & at risk for hypoglycemia. A1c targets must be individualized.

d: Postprandial glucose may be targeted if A1c goals are not met despite reaching preprandial glucose goals. Measurements should be made 1 to 2 hours after the beginning of a meal, generally represents peak levels.

e: Individualize goals based on shared decision making, cardiovascular risk, potential adverse effects of medications & patient preferences. Less stringent goals may be considered for frail patients with complicated comorbidities or those who have adverse medication effects. More intensive goal (e.g., < 120/80 mmHg) should be considered for patients if this goal can be safely reached.

Updated by Jeanine P. Abrons, Molly Henry, Elisha Andreas, and Emma Piehl..

Type 2 Diabetes: Glycemic Control Approaches

Therapeutic Approach	When to Use						When to Consider Next Approach	Other Notes
1. Monotherapy	Entry A1c < 7.5%						• If A1c goal not achieved after ~ 3 months with treatment approach: proceed to use of 2-drug combination (Dual therapy)	• Use with lifestyle management (including Medically Assisted Weight Loss)
	Consideration Area	**Specifics to Drug/Approach**						
	Efficacy	• High						
	Hypoglycemia risk	• Low						
	Associated weight impact	• Neutral/loss						
	Notable side effects	• Gastrointestinal (GI)/lactic acidosis						
	Costs	• Low						
2. Dual Therapy (Metformin or other 1st-line agent + additional medication)	Consider as an initial approach when A1c ≥ 7.5 to 9% or in patients with newly diagnosed type 2 diabetes who have A1c ≥ 1.5% above their glycemic target.						• If A1c goal not achieved after ~ 3 months with treatment approach: proceed to use of 3-drug combination (Triple therapy)	• Choice of additional medication dependent upon patient/disease-specific factors • Use with lifestyle management (including Medically Assisted Weight Loss)
	Drug Class	**Efficacy**	**Hypoglycemia Risk**	**Associated Weight Impact**	**Notable Side Effects**	**Costs**		
	Sulfonylureas	High	Moderate	Gain	Hypoglycemia	Low		
	Thiazolidinediones	High	Low	Gain	Edema, HF	Low		
	DPP-4 inhibitors	Intermediate	Low	Neutral	Rare	High		
	SGLT2 inhibitors	Intermediate	Low	Loss	GU, dehydration	High		
	GLP-1 receptor agonist	High	Low	Loss	GI	High		
	Insulin (Basal)	Highest	High	Gain	Hypoglycemia	High		

Notes: HF = heart failure; GU = genitourinary; GI = gastrointestinal.

When selecting a regimen, key patient factors should be considered, including (a) co-morbidities, (b) risk of hypoglycemia, (c) effects on body mass, (d) side effects, (e) costs, and (f) patient preferences Order of medications represents the order of recommended use

Based upon: AACE Comprehensive Type 2 Diabetes Management Algorithm (2020)—EXECUTIVE SUMMARY. https://pro.aace.com/disease-state-resources/diabetes/clinical-practice-guidelines-treatment-algorithms/comprehensive (Accessed 2022)

Prepared by Jeanine Abrons and Elisha Andreas

Type 2 Diabetes: Glycemic Control Approaches *(continued)*

Therapeutic Approach	When to Use	When to Consider Next Approach	Other Notes
3. Triple Therapy (Metformin or other 1st-line agent + 2nd-line agent + an additional medication)	Consider as an initial approach when A1c ≥ 7.5 to 9 <table><tr><th>Thiazolidinediones +</th><th>DPP-4 Inhibitor +</th><th>SGLT2 Inhibitors +</th><th>GLP-1 Receptor Agonist +</th><th>Insulin (Basal) +</th></tr><tr><td>SU</td><td>SU</td><td>SU</td><td>SU</td><td>TZD</td></tr><tr><td colspan="5">May select any 1 agent below to use in combination with 1st row</td></tr><tr><td>DPP-4-I</td><td>TZD</td><td>TZD</td><td>TZD</td><td>DPP-4-I</td></tr><tr><td>SGLT2-I</td><td>SGLT2-I</td><td>DPP-4-I</td><td>SGLT2-I</td><td>SGLT2-I</td></tr><tr><td>GLP-1-RA</td><td>Insulin</td><td>GLP-1-RA</td><td>Insulin</td><td>GLP-1-RA</td></tr><tr><td>Insulin</td><td></td><td>Insulin</td><td></td><td></td></tr></table>	If A1c goal not achieved after ~ 3 months with treatment approach * patient (1) on oral combo, move to insulin (basal) or GLP-1-RA, (2) on GLP-1-RA + insulin (basal), or (3) on optimal insulin (basal) + GLP-1-RA or mealtime insulin Maintain metformin with change while other oral agents may be discontinued	Choice of additional medication dependent upon patient/disease-specific factors Use with lifestyle management (including Medically Assisted Weight Loss)
4. Add or Intensify Insulin (Please see an insulin management algorithm)	Consider as an initial approach with A1c ≥ 10%, blood glucose ≥ 300 mg/dL OR patient is markedly symptomatic		
Entry A1c > 9	With no symptoms: Dual therapy or triple therapy With symptoms: Insulin + other agents		

Notes: HF = heart failure; GU = genitourinary; TZD = thiazolidinediones; DPP-4-I = DPP-4 inhibitors; SGLT2-I = SGLT2 inhibitors; GLP-1—RA; SU = sulfonylureas.

Based on glycemic control algorithm by AACE

Prepared by Jeanine Abrons and Elisha Andreas

Medications for Type 2 Diabetes

Drug Class	Primary Mechanism	Sample Medications (Generic/Brand)	Cost	Side Effects	Notes
Alpha glucosidase inhibitors	Blocks enzymes that break down starches in the intestines	Acarbose (Precose®), Miglitol (Glyset®)	Moderate	Bloating; gas; flatus	Oral A1c change: 0.5 to 1% Weight change: Minimal
Amylin	Slows food moving in the stomach	Pramlintide (Symlin®)	High	Nausea; vomiting; headache	Injected A1c change: 0.4 to 0.7% Weight change: Weight loss
Biguanides	↓ amount of glucose produced by the liver	Metformin (Glucophage®); Metformin XR (Glucophage® XR); Glumetza, Fortamet®)	Low	Indigestion; nausea, diarrhea (with higher doses)	Oral A1c change: 1 to 2% Weight change: No Risk for hypoglycemia: No
Bile acid sequestrants	↓ LDL cholesterol & blood glucose levels	Colesevelam (Welchol®)	High	Fainting, watery discharge; numbness/tingling/pain with cold weather; black/tarry stools; bloody vomit	Oral A1c change: 0.3 to 0.5% Weight change: No
Dopamine-2 Agonists	Helps ↓ blood glucose levels after a meal	Bromocriptine (Cycloset® or Parlodel®)	Moderate	Nausea, sleep	Oral A1c change: 0.6 to 0.9% Weight change: No
DPP-4-inhibitors	Slow the inactivation of GLP-1, a compound in the body that ↓ blood glucose levels	Alogliptin (Nesina®); Linagliptin (Tradjenta®); Saxagliptin (Onglyza®); Sitagliptin (Januvia®); Sitagliptin & metformin (Janumet®); Sitagliptin & metformin extended release (Janumet® XR)	High	Headache; nose & sinus congestion	Oral A1c change: 0.6 to 1.5% Weight change: No Risk of hypoglycemia: No

Medications for Type 2 Diabetes *(continued)*

Drug Class	Primary Mechanism	Sample Medications (Generic/Brand)	Cost	Side Effects	Notes
GLP-1 receptor agonists	Helps release insulin when blood glucose is high & lowers the amount of glucose made by the liver	Albiglutide (Eperzan®/Tanzeum®); Dulaglutide (Trulicity®); Exenatide (Byetta®); Exenatide extended release (Bydureon®); Liraglutide (Victoza®); Semaglutide (Ozempic®); Lixisenatide (Adlyxin)	High	Class effect: Nausea/vomiting/diarrhea; injection site pain Exenatide: Headache; hypoglycemia Liraglutide: Tachycardia; headache; constipation	Injected; Exception = semaglutide (oral GLP-1 agonist) A1c change: 1 to 1.5% Weight loss: 3 to 6 lbs Black box warnings: Dulaglutide, Exenatide, & Semaglutide (risk of thyroid C-cell tumors
Meglitinides	Helps beta cells of the pancreas release more insulin	Nateglinide (Starlix®); Repaglinide (Prandin®)	Moderate	Hypoglycemia; weight gain; GI disturbances	Oral A1c change: 0.8 to 1.5% Weight change: Gain 1.5 to 4 pounds
SGL2 inhibitors	Blocks glucose from being reabsorbed by the kidneys	Canagliflozin (Invokana®); Dapagliflozin (Farxiga®); Empagliflozin (Jardiance®); Ertugliflozin (Steglatro)	High	Yeast infections & urinary tract infections; colds	Oral A1c change: 0.5 to 1% Weight loss: 1 to 4 lbs Risk of hypoglycemia: No
Sulfonylureas	Helps beta cells of the pancreas release more insulin	Glimepiride (Amaryl); Glipizide (Glucotrol); Glipizide extended release (Glucotrol XL); Glyburide (Diabeta)	Low	Hypoglycemia; weight gain; nausea	Oral A1c change: 1 to 2% Weight gain: 2 to 3 lbs
Thiazolidinediones (TZDs)	Helps insulin work better in muscles/fat cells; ↓ glucose production in the liver	Pioglitazone (Actos); Rosiglitazone (Avandia)	Low	Swelling; change to LDL cholesterol	Oral A1c change: 1 to 2% Weight gain: 2 to 6 lbs Risk of hypoglycemia: No

References: American Diabetes Association Medications. http://main.diabetes.org/dforg/pdfs/2019/2019-cg-medications.pdf. Accessed November 2021. American Association of Nurse Practitioners. Diabetes Medications. https://storage.aarp.org/www/documents/education/Patients-Diabetes-Medication-Table-2020.pdf. Accessed November 2021.

Insulin and Insulin Analogues

Type	Generic Name (Trade Name)	Onset (hours)	Peak (hours)	Duration (hours)	Administration Notes
Ultra Rapid Acting					
Analogue	Aspart (Fiasp®)*	0.25 to 4	1 to 2.5	5 to 7	• Give at start of meal or within 20 minutes of start
Rapid Acting					
Analogue	Aspart (Novolog®)***	0.2 to 0.5	1 to 3	3 to 7	• Give Novolog right before meals (within 5–10 minutes)
	Glulisine (Apidra®)**	0.2 to 0.5	0.6 to 2	3 to 4	• Give Apidra within 15 minutes before a meal or within 20 minutes after start of meal
	Lispro (Humalog®, Admelog®)**	0.5 to 0.75	2.4 to 2.8	5.7 to 6.6	• Give Lispro within 15 minutes before or right after a meal
Short Acting					
Human	Regular (Humulin R®, Novolin®)**	~0.5	0.5 to 2.5	~8	• Give 30 minutes before meal
	Regular U-500 (Humulin R® Concentrated)**	< 0.25	0.5 to 0.8	13 to 24	SC [Injection/CSII]
Intermediate Acting					
Human	NPH (Humulin-N®, Novolin-N®)*	1 to 2	4 to 12	14 to 24	• Dosed once or twice daily
Long Acting					
Analogue; Human	Degludec (Tresiba®)*	~1	~9	Not applicable	• Typically given once daily at bedtime or twice daily
	Detemir (Levemir®) *	3 to 4	3 to 9	6 to 23	
	Glargine (Lantus®)*		~10 to 12	10.8 to > 24	
	Glargine (Basaglar®)*		~12	≥ 24	
	Glargine (Toujeo®)*	6	~12 to 16		
Insulin Combinations					
Combination	Degludec + Aspart (Ryzodeg® 70/30)*	0.23	1.2	> 24	
	NPH + Regular (Humulin® 70/30; Novolin® 70/30)*	0.5	2 to 12	18 to 24	
	Lispro protamine + Lispro (Humalog® Mix 50/50; Humalog® Mix 75/25)*	0.25 to 0.5	50/50 Mix: 0.8 to 48 75/25 Mix: 1 to 6.5	14 to 24	
	Aspart protamine + Aspart (Novolog® Mix 70/30)*	0.17 to 0.33	1 to 4	18 to 24	
	Glargine + GLP-1 Agonist (Soliqua® 100/33)*	See individual drugs	2.5 to 3	T½ = 3 h; Clearance = 35 L/h	
	Degludec + GLP-1 Agonist (Xultophy® 100/3.6)*		Not applicable	> 24	

Note: * = Administration route = SC; ** = Administration route = SC/CSII; CSII = continuous subcutaneous insulin infusion; GLP = glucagon-like peptide; SC = subcutaneous injection.

To add basal (Long-acting) insulin: for A1c < 8% with total daily dose (TDD) of 0.1 to 0.2 U/kg or for A1c > 8% TDD of 0.2 to 0.3 U/kg. Titrate to glycemic goals every 2 to 3 days

To intensify insulin (prandial control): Add a GLP1 receptor antagonist or SGLT2i or DPP4i: Then add prandial insulin: 1) begin prandial before largest meal. If not at goal, increase arrow to before 2 or 3 meals (start at 10% of basal dose or 5 units), OR 2) Begin prandial insulin before each meal (50% Basal/50% prandial TDD = 0.3/0.5 U/kg)

Updated by Jeanine P. Abrons and Emma Piehl

Asthma: Definition & Diagnosis— Based on the 2021 GINA Guidelines

Definition of Asthma: Chronic airway inflammation with a history of typical respiratory symptoms such as wheezing, shortness of breath, chest tightness, and cough that varies over time and intensity, together with variable expiratory airflow limitation.

Factors that trigger or worsen Asthma:
- Viral infections
- Tobacco smoke
- Exercise
- Stress
- Allergens *(e.g., dust mites, pollens, cockroaches)*

Asthma Diagnosis Features:

History of Variable Respiratory Symptoms		Evidence of Variable Expiratory Airway Limitation		Consider Other Contexts
• Often > typical symptoms • Variability in timing/intensity • Often occur/are worse at night or with waking • Often triggered by exercise, laughter, allergens, or cold air • Occur with or worsen with viral infections	PLUS	• FEV1/FVC ratio < normal at least once • Variation in lung function is > than in healthy people *(e.g., significant bronchodilator responsiveness or reversibility, average daily diurnal PEF variability > 10% (13% in kids); FEV increases by > 12% after 4 weeks of anti-inflammatory treatment)**	PLUS	• Using controller medication • Occupation or work aggravated asthma • Pregnant women • Elderly • Smokers/ex-smokers • Persistent cough as only symptom

* > variation or more times seen = more confidence in diagnosis; testing may need to be repeated during symptoms; significant bronchodilator reversibility may be absent during severe exacerbations or viral infections; see GINA 2021, Chapter 1

What to Assess in Asthma:
- Symptom & exacerbation control over 4 weeks
- Modifiable risk factors
- Lung function (before treatment; 3 to 6 months later; periodically)
- Comorbidities: Gastroesophageal reflux disease; obesity; obstructive sleep apnea; depression; anxiety
- Treatment issues (e.g., side effects; inhaler technique; asthma action plan; goals/preferences)
- Confirm diagnosis is correct.
- Personalization/adjustment of therapy based on continual cycle of assessment, treatment & review to minimize symptoms & exacerbations.

Cards by Haley Morrison and Jeanine P. Abrons; updated by Jeanine P. Abrons

Asthma: Assessment of Level of Control— Based on the 2021 GINA Guidelines

Assessment of Level of Control

Uncontrolled	Partly Controlled	Well Controlled
• 3 or 4 of the criteria listed below	• 1 to 2 of the criteria listed below	• None of the criteria below

Criteria:
- Daytime symptoms more than twice/week
- Any night waking due to asthma
- Short-acting beta agonist (SABA) reliever needed more than twice/week
- Any activity limitation due to asthma

Based on Box 2-2 of the GINA 2021 Guidelines

Risk Factors for Poor Asthma Outcomes:

Risk Factors for Exacerbations		
Medications	• Inadequate or inhaled corticosteroids not prescribed	• Incorrect inhaler technique
	• Poor adherence	• High SABA use
Other Medical Conditions	• Chronic rhinosinusitis	• Confirmed food allergy
	• Obesity	• GERD
	• Pregnancy	
Context	• Major socioeconomic challenges	
Lung Function	• Low FEV1 (especially if < 60% predicted; higher reversibility)	
Other Tests	• Blood eosinophilia; elevated FeNO in allergic adults on inhaled corticosteroids	
Other Major Independent Risk Factors	• Previous history of intubation • Previous history of intensive care for asthma • ≥ 1 severe exacerbations in the last 12 months	
Exposures	Smoking, allergen exposure, air pollution	
Risk Factors for Developing Fixed Airflow Limitation		

- Preterm birth, low birth weight, > infant weight gain
- Medications: Lack of inhaled corticosteroid (ICS) treatments in patients who had severe exacerbation
- Exposures: tobacco smoke; noxious chemicals; occupational exposures
- Low FEV1
- Chronic mucus hypersecretion
- Sputum or blood eosinophilia

Based on Box 2-2 of 2021 GINA Guidelines

Cards by Haley Morrison and Jeanine P. Abrons; updated by Jeanine P. Abrons

Initial Asthma Treatment Steps and Recommended Options for Adults and Adolescents Based on the 2021 GINA Guidelines

Presenting Symptoms	Preferred Initial Treatment	Alternative Initial Treatment	Before Starting Initial Controller Treatment	After Starting Initial Controller Treatment
Infrequent asthma symptoms (< twice per month & no risk factors for exacerbations)	Inhaled low dose corticosteroid (ICS)-formoterol as needed	Low-dose ICS taken whenever SABA is taken in combination or separate inhalers	• Record evidence for diangosis of asthma • Record patient's symptom control & risk factors/lung function • Consider factors impacting initial treatement options (e.g., adherence with control) • Check patient inhaler technique • Schedule follow-up visit	• Review patient response based on urgency or every 2 to 3 months • Check adherence and inhaler technique frequently • Step down treatment once control has been maintained for 3 months
Asthma symptoms or need for a reliever twice a month or more	Inhaled low-dose ICS-formoterol as needed	Low-dose ICS taken with as-needed SABA; consider likely adherence with daily ICS		
Troublesome asthma symptoms most days; or waking due to asthma once a week or more, especially if any risk factors exist	Low dose ICS-formoterol maintenance and reliever therapy	Low dose ICS-LABA with as-needed SABA OR medium-dose ICS with as-needed SABA; consider likely adherence with daily controller		
Initial asthma presentation is with severely uncontrolled asthma or with an acute exacerbation	Medium-dose ICS-formoterol maintenance and reliever therapy	**Alternative:** High-dose ICS **Additional:** Tiotropium or LTRA		

Based upon GINA Pocket Guidelines 2021 page 24: https://ginasthma.org/pocket-guide-for-asthma-management-and-prevention/ (Accessed 2021)

Cards by Haley Morrison and Jeanine P. Abrons

Selecting Initial Controller Treatment in Children Ages 6 to 11 with a Diagnosis of Asthma— Based on the 2021 GINA Guidelines

Step	Preferred Controller	Alternative or Additional Controller	Preferred Reliever	Alternative Reliever
1	Low-dose ICS taken whenever SABA taken	**Alternative:** Consider daily low-dose ICS	SABA as needed	Low-dose ICS-formoterol reliever for maintenance and relief
2	Daily low-dose ICS	**Alternative:** Daily LTRA OR low-dose ICS taken whenever SABA taken		
3	Low-dose ICS + LABA OR medium-dose ICS OR very low-dose ICS-formoterol maintenance and reliever	**Alternative:** Low-dose ICS + LTRA		
4	Medium-dose ICS + LABA OR low-dose ICS-formoterol maintenance and reliever therapy; refer for expert advice	**Alternative:** High-dose ICS + LABA **Additional:** Tiotropium OR LTRA		
5	Refer for phenotypic assessment +/- higher-dose ICS-LABA or add-on therapy, e.g., anti-IgE	**Additional:** Add on anti-IL5 OR add-on low-dose OCS, but consider side effects		

ICS = Inhaled corticosteroid; SABA = short-acting bronchodilator; LTRA = leukotriene receptor antagonist; OCS = oral corticosteroid; IL5 = Interleukin-5

Personalized Asthma Management Continuous Cycle

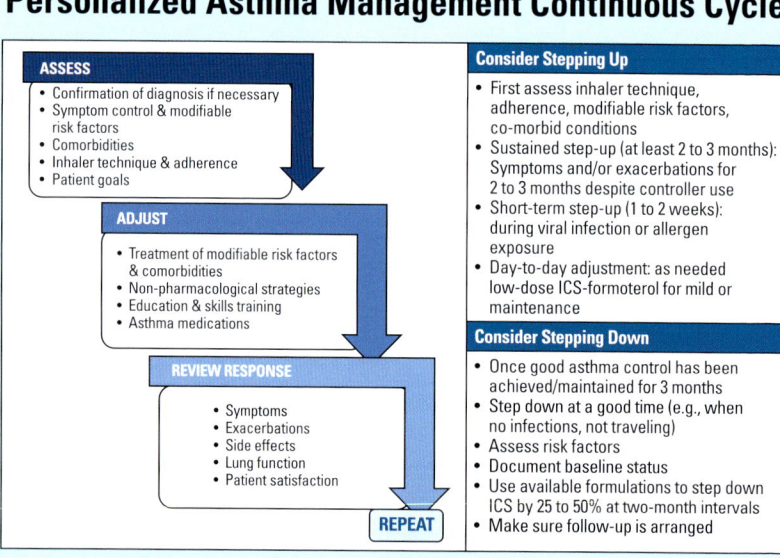

ASSESS
- Confirmation of diagnosis if necessary
- Symptom control & modifiable risk factors
- Comorbidities
- Inhaler technique & adherence
- Patient goals

ADJUST
- Treatment of modifiable risk factors & comorbidities
- Non-pharmacological strategies
- Education & skills training
- Asthma medications

REVIEW RESPONSE
- Symptoms
- Exacerbations
- Side effects
- Lung function
- Patient satisfaction

REPEAT

Consider Stepping Up
- First assess inhaler technique, adherence, modifiable risk factors, co-morbid conditions
- Sustained step-up (at least 2 to 3 months): Symptoms and/or exacerbations for 2 to 3 months despite controller use
- Short-term step-up (1 to 2 weeks): during viral infection or allergen exposure
- Day-to-day adjustment: as needed low-dose ICS-formoterol for mild or maintenance

Consider Stepping Down
- Once good asthma control has been achieved/maintained for 3 months
- Step down at a good time (e.g., when no infections, not traveling)
- Assess risk factors
- Document baseline status
- Use available formulations to step down ICS by 25 to 50% at two-month intervals
- Make sure follow-up is arranged

Cards by Haley Morrison and Jeanine P. Abrons; updated by Jeanine P. Abrons

Suggested Low, Medium, and High Dosing of Inhaled Corticosteroids in Asthma

Steroid Daily Dosing	LOW-Dose Inhaled Corticosteroid (in Mcg)		MEDIUM-Dose Inhaled Corticosteroid (in Mcg)		HIGH-Dose Inhaled Corticosteroid (in Mcg)	
Drug/Age Category	Children 6 to 11 Years	Adults and Adolescents	Children 6 to 11 Years	Adults and Adolescents	Children 6 to 11 Years	Adults and Adolescents
BDP (pMDI, HFA)	100 to 200	200 to 500	> 200 to 400	> 500 to 1,000	> 400	> 1000
BDP (pMDI, extrafine particle, HFA)	50 to 100	100 to 200	> 100 to 200	> 200 to 400	> 200	> 400
Budesonide (DPI)	100 to 200	200 to 400	> 200 to 400	> 400 to 800	> 400	> 800
Budesonide nebules	250 to 500	Not applicable (N/A)	> 500 to 1000	N/A	> 1000	N/A
Ciclesonide (pMDI, extrafine particle, HFA)	80	80 to 160	> 80 to 160	> 160 to 320	> 160	> 320
Fluticasone furoate (DPI)	50	100	50	100	N/A	200
Fluticasone propionate (DPI)	50 to 100	100 to 250	> 100 to 200	> 250 to 500	> 200	> 500
Fluticasone propionate (pMDI, HFA)	50 to 100	100 to 250	> 100 to 200	> 250 to 500	> 200	> 500
Mometasone furoate (DPI)	N/A	200	N/A	200	N/A	400
Mometasone Furoate (pMDI, HFA)	100	200 to 400	100	200 to 400	200	400

Beclomethasone Dipropionate = BDP; pMDI = pressurized metered dose inhaler; HFA = hydrofluoroalkane propellant (non-CFC); DPI = dry powdered inhaler

Cards by Haley Morrison and Jeanine P. Abrons

Assessment of Airflow Limitation/Symptoms in Chronic Obstructive Pulmonary Disease (COPD)

COPD Airflow Limitation			Symptom (Dyspnea)	
GOLD Class	**Degree of Limitation**	**FEV₁****	**mMRC Grade****	**Description of Limitation**
1	Mild	$FEV_1 \geq 80\%$ predicted	0	Only gets breathless with strenuous activity
2	Moderate	50 to $79\% \leq FEV_1$ predicted	1	Gets short of breath when hurrying on level ground or walking slightly uphill
3	Severe	30 to $49\% \leq FEV_1$ predicted	2	Walks slower than others of age on level ground due to breathlessness or has to stop for breath when walking at own pace on level ground
4	Very severe	$FEV_1 < 30\%$ predicted	3	Stops for breath when walking ~ 100 meters or after a few minutes walking on level ground
			4	Too breathless to leave house or when dressing or undressing
			CAT Element	**Description of Limitation**
			Cough	Never (0) to All the time (5)
			Phlegm (Mucus)	None in chest (0) to Completely full of phlegm (5)
			Chest tightness	Not tight at all (0) to Very tight (5)
			Hill or 1 Flight of Stairs	Not breathless while walking (0) to Very breathless while walking (5)
			Limits activity at home	Not limited (0) to Very limited (5)
			Confidence leaving home	Confident (0) to Not confident (5)
			Sleeping	Sleep soundly (0) to Don't sleep soundly (5)
			Energy	Have lots (0) to No energy at all (5)

** *Forced expiratory volume; Correlation between FEV1, symptoms, & health status impairment is weak. Formal symptom assessment also required. Spirometric cut-points are for simplicity. To ↓ variability, perform spirometry after ≥ 1 dose of short-acting inhaled bronchodilator*

*** *mMRC: modified British Medical Research Council;* ^CAT: COPD Assessment Test;

Notes: *Post-bronchodilator FEV1/FVC < 0.70 confirms airflow limitation;*

References: *CAT = Jones et al. ERJ 2009; 34(3):648–54; mMRC = CM Fletcher, BMJ 1960; 2020 GOLD Guidelines available at: https://goldcopd.org/wp-content/uploads/2020/03/GOLD-2020-POCKET-GUIDE-ver1.0_FINAL-WMV.pdf (Accessed October 2020)*

Use these assessments to determine ABCD Groups in COPD.

Reference: From the Global Strategy for Diagnosis, Management and Prevention of COPD 2022©.

Prepared by Jeanine P. Abrons and Anh Luong

Assessment to Determine ABCD Groups in Chronic Obstructive Pulmonary Disease (COPD)

STEP 1: Confirm Diagnosis

- Use spirometry to define grade (airflow limits)
- Post-bronchodilator $FEV_1/FVC < 0.70$ confirms airflow limitation

With Presence of Key Indicators:
- Dyspnea *(progressive; worse with exercise; persistent)*
- Chronic cough *(intermittent; unproductive; recurrent wheeze)*
- Chronic sputum
- Recurrent lower respiratory tract infections
- Family history

STEP 2: Assess Airflow Limitation/Symptom Severity

- Classify airflow limitation severity (GOLD 1 to 4)
- Assess symptoms (use mMRC Scale & CAT Assessment)

Class	Description
Low Severity	• $mMRC \leq 1$ **OR** • $CAT \leq 9$
High Severity	• $mMRC \geq 2$ **OR** • $CAT \geq 10$

STEP 3: Exacerbation History

- Prior exacerbation prevalence/severity
- # of prior hospitalizations/exacerbation risk

Class	Description
Low Risk	• 0 or 1 exacerbation (not leading to hospital admission in last 12 months)
High Risk	• 1 or ≥ 2 exacerbations resulting in hospital admission in past 12 months

STEP 4: Combine Symptom Assessment/Exacerbation Risk

- Assessment of symptoms/risk of exacerbation

GOLD Group	Description
A	• Low symptom severity • Low exacerbation risk
B	• High symptom severity • Low exacerbation risk
C	• Low symptom severity • High exacerbation risk
D	• High symptom severity • High exacerbation risk

Reference: 2021 GOLD Guidelines available at: https://goldcopd.org/wp-content/uploads/2020/03/GOLD-2020-POCKET-GUIDE-ver1.0_FINAL-WMV.pdf (Accessed 2022)

Card by Anh Luong and Jeanine P. Abrons

Initial Therapies Based on Symptom Severity/Exacerbation Risk for COPD

Group	Group Description	Recommended Therapies
A	**"Low symptom severity/Low exacerbation risk"** 0 or 1 exacerbation in past year not leading to hospital admission & mMRC of 0 to 1 &/or CAT < 10	• **Preferred Treatment:** Initial: Either a short- or long-acting bronchodilator • If no improvements to initial therapy: stop / try alternative bronchodilator
B	**"High symptom severity/Low exacerbation risk"** 0 or 1 exacerbation in past year not leading to hospital admission & mMRC ≥ 2 &/or CAT ≥ 10	• **Preferred Treatment:** Initial: Long-acting bronchodilator monotherapy (LABA or LAMA) ○ If symptoms persist on monotherapy or severe breathlessness: use 2 bronchodilators (LABA + LAMA) for initial therapy • No evidence to recommend one class of long-acting bronchodilators over another for initial treatment. Choice will depend on patient's perception of symptom relief.
C	**"Low symptom severity/High exacerbation risk"** ≥ 1 exacerbation with hospital admission in past year or ≥ 2 exacerbations & mMRC of 0 to 1 &/or CAT < 10	• **Preferred Treatment:** Initial: Long-acting bronchodilator monotherapy (LAMA superior)

D	**"High symptom severity/High exacerbation risk"** ≥ 2 or ≥ 1 leading to hospital admission in past year & mMRC ≥ 2 &/or CAT ≥ 10	• **Preferred Treatment:** Initial: LAMA
		  ○ Severe symptoms (CAT ≥ 20), especially with dyspnea/exercise limitation: LAMA/LABA
		  ○ COPD + asthma history &/or eosinophil counts ≥ 300 cells/microliter: consider LABA/ICS
		    – Use as initial therapy only after considering risks vs. benefits of ICS due to potential side effects from ICS (i.e., pneumonia)

Non-Pharmacological Treatment for A, B, C, D: smoking cessation (no recommendation made for e-cigarette use for smoking cessation); maintain or increase physical activity; flu/pneumococcal vaccine; CDC recommends Tdap (dTaP/dTPa) vaccine for adults not vaccinated in adolescence for protection against pertussis (whooping cough)

Note: For all recommendations listed, escalate or de-escalate depending on patient's response. Continue current treatment if there is symptomatic benefit. Discontinue or try alternative treatment class if no symptomatic benefit. 2022 GOLD Guidelines available at: hhttps://goldcopd.org/2022-gold-reports/ (iAccessed 2021)

Card by Anh Luong and Jeanine P. Abrons

COPD Follow-Up

1. If response to initial treatment is appropriate, maintain it.
2. If not:

• Consider the predominant treatable trait to target (dyspnea or exacerbations) • If both need to be targeted, follow management for exacerbations	• Place patient in box corresponding to current treatment & follow indications
• Assess response, adjust & review	• Recommendations don't depend on ABCD assessment at diagnosis

COPD Exacerbation Management (Severe but not Life-Threatening)

Bronchodilators +/– short-acting anticholinergics recommended as initial bronchodilators in acute	• Increase doses &/or frequency of SABDs • Combine SABA + anticholinergics • Consider LABDs when patient becomes stable	
Oral Corticosteroids For 5 to 7 days	• Prednisone 40 mg daily x 5 days recommended • Oral/IV prednisolone equally effective • Studies suggest glucocorticoids may have less benefit in those with lower levels of blood eosinophils	
Nebulized budesonide alone	• IV methylprednisolone alternative	
Antibiotics For 5 to 7 days	• 3 cardinal symptoms: ↑ in dyspnea, sputum volume & sputum purulence • 2 cardinal symptoms: if 1 or 2 symptoms is ↑ in sputum purulence or mechanical ventilation required	• Antibiotic choice should be based on local antibiogram • Typical empiric treatment: aminopenicillin + clavulanic acid, macrolide or tetracycline • If exacerbations are often, airflow limitation is severe &/or mechanical ventilation is required: potential for resistant pathogens or gram-negative bacteria not sensitive to typical empiric treatment

In all cases: Enforce smoking cessation; use venous thromboembolism prophylaxis if not contraindicated: SQ heparin or low molecular weight heparin & identify/treatment comorbidities (e.g., heart failure, arrhythmias, pulmonary embolism, etc.) SABD = short-acting bronchodilators; SABA = short-acting beta-agonists. LABD = long-acting beta-agonists.

COVID-19 in Patients with COPD

Maintenance Treatment During COVID-19 Pandemic	• Continue maintenance therapy, including ICS (no support for changing regimen to ↓ risk of COVID-19)
COVID-19 Treatment in COPD	• Treat COVID-19 & COPD • Systemic steroids ok (no data this modifies susceptibility to COVID-19 or worsens outcomes)
COVID-19 Patients With COPD Exacerbations	• Systemic steroids ok (no data this modifies susceptibility to COVID-19 or worsens outcomes) • If bacterial co-infections, use broad-spectrum antibiotics
Other considerations	• If possible, use meter dose inhalers (MDIs), dry powder inhalers (DPIs), &/or soft mist inhalers (SMI) instead of nebulizers (nebulizers carry risk of more contaminated aerosol/droplets produced)

Common Maintenance Medications Used in COPD

Drug (Generic)	Inhaler Type	Nebulizer (Yes/No)	Duration of Action (hours)
Beta2-Agonists			
Short-Acting (SABA)			
Albuterol (Salbutamol)	MDI & DPI	Y	4 to 6; 12 (extended release)
Levalbuterol	MDI	Y	6 to 8
Fenoterol	MDI	Y	4 to 6
Terbutaline	DPI	N	
Long-Acting (LABA)			
Arformoterol		Y	12
Formoterol	DPI	Y	12
Indacaterol	DPI	N	24
Olodaterol	SMI	N	24
Salmeterol	MDI & DPI	N	12
Anticholinergics			
Short-Acting (SAMA)			
Ipratropium bromide	MDI	Y	6 to 8
Oxitropium bromide	MDI	Y	7 to 9
Long-Acting Muscarinic Agonist (LAMA)			
Aclidinium bromide	DPI, MDI	N	12
Glycopyrronium bromide	DPI	Y	12 to 24
Tiotropium	DPI, SMI, MDI	N	24
Umeclidinium	DPI	N	24
Glycopyrrolate	DPI	Y	12
Revefenacin	Nebulizer only	Y	24

MDI = Meter dose inhaler; DPI = Dry powder inhaler; SMI = Soft mist inhaler

Card by Anh Luong and Jeanine P. Abrons

Common Maintenance Medications Used in COPD *(continued)*

Drug (Generic)	Inhaler Type	Nebulizer (Yes/No)	Duration of Action (hours)
SABA + SAMA			
Albuterol (Salbutamol) + ipratropium	SMI, MDI	Y	6 to 8
Fenoterol + ipratropium	SMI	Y	6 to 8
LABA + LAMA			
Formoterol + aclidinium	DPI	N	12
Formoterol + glycopyrronium	MDI	N	12
Indacaterol + glycopyrrolate	DPI	N	12 to 24
Vilanterol + umeclidinium	DPI	N	24
Olodaterol + tiotropium	SMI	N	24
LABA + ICS			
Formoterol + beclometasone	MDI, DPI	N	12
Formoterol + budesonide	MDI, DPI	N	12
Formoterol + mometasone	MDI	N	12
Salmeterol + fluticasone	MDI, DPI	N	12
Vilanterol + fluticasone furoate	DPI	N	24
LABA + LAMA + ICS			
Vilanterol + umeclidinium + fluticasone	DPI	N	24
Formoterol + glycopyrronium + beclometasone	MDI	N	12

Medication/Medication Type	Formulation	Duration of Action (hours)
Methylxanthines		
Aminophylline	IV solution	Variable, but up to 24 hours
Theophylline (SR)	Solution, tablet	Variable, but up to 24 hours
Phosphodiesterase-4 Inhibitors (PDE-4 Inhibitors)		
Roflumilast	Tablet	24 hours

MDI = Meter dose inhaler; DPI = Dry powder inhaler; SMI = Soft mist inhaler

Card by Anh Luong and Jeanine P. Abrons

Testing for COVID-19

For the most updated information on COVID-19, please visit https://www.cdc.gov/coronavirus/2019-ncov/.

To Test or Not to Test? Sample Scenarios	Should Testing Occur & When
Known Symptoms	• Yes; Test as soon as possible
Known exposure to someone suspected or known to have COVID-19	• Fully vaccinated: Yes; Test 3 to 5 days after exposure • Not fully vaccinated: Yes; Test immediately & again in 5 to 7 days if initial test was negative
Not vaccinated	• Test as soon as possible
Individuals who have tested positive within the past 3 months	• No new symptoms: Testing not required • New symptoms: Test as soon as possible

Specimen Type

Type of Testing	Serology Test	Recommended Use	Processing Time
Viral Testing Antigen tests*: detects antigen NAATs**: detects RNA	• NAATs: nasopharyngeal, nasal mid-turbinate, anterior nasal, or saliva • Antigen: nasopharyngeal or anterior nasal	• To diagnose acute (or current) infection in symptomatic/asymptomatic individuals	• NAATs processed in a lab: ~1–3 days • NAATs processed at POC: 15–45 minutes • Antigen tests: 15 minutes
Antibody or Serology Testing (not FDA authorized; not CDC recommended as sole basis for diagnosis)	• Blood sample that detects antibodies spike in glycoprotein (S) and nucleocapsid hosphoprotein (N)	• To determine if individuals were previously infected, even if no symptoms are present • To detect possible immunity • In conjunction with viral tests to support clinical assessment in late illness • Suspicion of post-infectious syndrome • Not recommended to assess immunity after vaccination	• Binding Ab detection: 30 minutes in a field setting, hours in a laboratory • Neutralizing Ab detection: may take up to five days but these are not approved

- *Gold Standard testing = Nucleic acid amplification tests (NAATs), such as RT-PCR*
- *Antibody testing is approved by the FDA currently under emergency use authorization since November 2020.*
- *Viral tests are less sensitive than real-time reverse transcription-polymerase chain reaction (RT-PCR).*

*Antigen test is frequently referred to as "rapid test"
**NAAT (Nucleic Acid Amplification Tests) include molecular, PCR, and viral RNA tests

Card by Shushanna Galstyan and Jeanine P. Abrons; updated by Michael Parisi Mercado

Collecting, Handling, and Testing of Clinical Specimens for COVID-19

CDC-Recommended Specimen Types for Initial Diagnosis*	Testing Technique for Accurate Results	Safe Handling / Collection of Specimens	Respiratory Specimens
• A nasopharyngeal (NP) specimen • An oropharyngeal (OP) specimen • A nasal mid-turbinate swab (using a flocked tapered swab) • An anterior nares (nasal swab) specimen (using a flocked or spun polyester swab) • Nasopharyngeal wash/aspirate or nasal wash/aspirate (NW) specimen • A saliva specimen	• Immediately place sterile swabs into transport tube containing 2 to 3 mL of either viral transport medium (VTM), Amies transport medium, or sterile saline (unless using a test analyzed directly—i.e., some point-of-care tests). • Immediately place specimens and non-bacteriostatic saline used to collect specimens into a sterile transport tube.	• When collecting specimens or within 6 feet of patients suspected to be infected with SARS-CoV-2, maintain proper infection control practice. ○ N95 or higher-level respirator (or face mask if respirator not available), eye protection, gloves, & gown. • Personnel handling specimens but not collecting and not working within six feet of the patient should follow standard precautions. It is recommended to wear a face mask at all times. • Insert minitip swab with flexible shaft (wire or plastic) in the nostril parallel to the palate (not upward) until resistance is encountered or the distance is equivalent to that from the ear to the nostril of the patient, indicating contact with the nasopharynx. • The swab should reach the depth equal to the distance from the nostrils to outer ear opening. • Leave the swab in place for several seconds to absorb secretions. • Gently rub & roll the swab. • Slowly remove the swab while rotating it. • Ensure minitip is saturated with fluid (specimens can be collected from both sides with the same swab, which is only needed if saturation not reached); consider if deviated septum or blockage creates difficulty in obtaining the specimen in one nostril.	• Ensure proper specimen to ensure avoidance of false negative results. • See CDC website for proper step-by-step specimen guidance. • Use only synthetic fiber swabs with a plastic/wire shaft. • CDC recommends only OP swabs—combine with a single tube to maximize test sensitivity and limit use of testing resources. • Do not use calcium alginate swabs or swabs with wooden shafts—these may contain substances that inactivate some viruses and inhibit molecular tests.

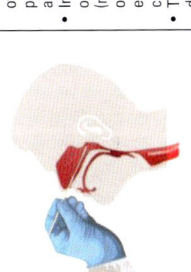

Testing lower respiratory tract specimens is also an option. For patients who develop a productive cough, sputum should be collected and tested for SARS-CoV-2. The induction of sputum is not recommended. When under certain clinical circumstances (e.g., those receiving invasive mechanical ventilation), a lower respiratory tract aspirate or bronchoalveolar lavage sample should be collected and tested as a lower respiratory tract specimen.

Card by Shushanna Galstyan and Jeanine P. Abrons; updated by Michael Parisi Mercado and Jeanine Abrons

Collecting Anterior Nasal Swab and Nasal Mid-Turbinate Specimens for COVID-19 Testing

Anterior Nasal Swab Sample Collection for COVID-19 Testing	*Nasal Mid-Turbinate Sample* Collection for COVID-19 Testing
Initial set-up prior to sample collection 1. Open the kit. 2. Apply hand sanitizer with at least 60% alcohol. **Collecting the sample** 3. Remove swab from container and be careful not to touch soft end with your hands. 4. Insert entire swab (no more than ¾ of an inch) into one nostril, ensuring you do not insert more than once into the nostril. 5. Slowly rotate the swab so that it rubs along the insides of the nostril for 15 seconds, getting as much nasal discharge as possible. 6. Gently remove the swab. 7. Repeat steps 4-6 in the other nostril, with the same end of the swab. **Preparing sample for return** 8. Place swab in sterile tube and snap off end of the tube at line, as this will allow the swab to fit in the tube; cap the tube and screw closed tightly so it doesn't leak. 9. Wash hands or reapply hand sanitizer. 10. Place tube in biohazard bag and seal it. **Returning the sample and cleaning up** 11. Hand the bag to testing personnel or follow instructions for returning. 12. Dispose of remaining testing items. 13. Wash hands or reapply hand sanitizer.	**Initial set-up prior to sample collection** 1. Disinfect surface where kit will be used, remove kit, and lay out contents of kit. Read instructions. 2. Wash hands with soap/water or use hand sanitizer if soap/ water not available. **Collecting the sample** 3. Remove swab from package and be careful to not touch soft end with your hands or anything else. 4. Insert entire swab straight back into nostril (less than one inch) until resistance is noted. 5. Slowly rotate the swab so that it rubs along the insides of nasal passage several times. 6. Gently remove the swab. 7. Repeat steps 4 to 6 in the other nostril, with the same end of the swab. **Preparing sample for return** 8. Place swab in sterile tube and snap off end of the tube at line, as this will allow the swab to fit in the tube; cap the tube and screw tightly so it doesn't leak. 9. Wash hands or reapply hand sanitizer. 10. Place tube in biohazard bag and seal it. **Returning the sample and cleaning up** 11. Hand the bag to testing personnel or follow instructions for returning. 12. Dispose of remaining testing items. 13. Wash hands or reapply hand sanitizer.

* Sample kits may vary; it is important to follow the instructions and to use materials included in your sample kit only.
* Use approved sample kits only.

Adapted from the CDC, last updated October 27, 2021. For the most updated information, please visit cdc.gov/coronavirus/2019-nCoV.

Community-Acquired Pneumonia (CAP) Management

Causative Bacteria		Respiratory Viruses	
Streptococcus pnemoniae	Chlamydophila pneumonia	Influenza A & B	Rhinoviruses
Haemophilus influenza	Legionella species	Parainfluenza viruses	Adenoviruses
Moraxella catarrhalis	Mycoplasma pneumonia	Respiratory syncytial virus	Human bocaviruses
Other gram (-) bacilli[a]	Staphylococcus aureus[a]		

Signs and Symptoms		Predisposing Risk Factors	
Pulmonary signs & symptoms (i.e., cough [with or without sputum production]; dyspnea; pleuritic chest pain; tachypnea; ↑ effort in breathing; crackles or rales; hypoxemia; sputum production)		Age > 65	Immunosupressive conditions
		Smoking	Alcoholism
		Viral respiratory tract infections	Chronic obstructive pulmonary disease (COPD)
Systemic signs & symptoms (i.e., fever; chills; fatigue; malaise; tachycardia)		Chronic comorbidities (chronic cardiovascular, or cerebrovascular disease, diabetes, and dementia)	Lung function changes (e.g., cystic fibrosis; Karagener syndrome; Young syndrome; immotile cilia syndrome; bioterrorism [anthrax; tularemia; plague])
Radiographic findings on chest X-ray (i.e., opacities; lobar consolidations; interstitial infiltrates)			

How Is CAP Diagnosed?	How Is the Severity of CAP Evaluated?
• Presence of clinically compatible signs/symptoms with radiographic findings • Blood cultures (x2) and/or expectorated sputum samples for culture & gram stain[*b] • Legionella & pneumococcal urinary assays[b]; Obtain serum procalcitonin level if culture results are negative	Can be made through either CURB-65 (see notes for criteria) or Pneumonia Severity Index (PSI; also known as the PORT score)

Note: Airways consider institution-specific susceptibilities; *C = confusion; U = urea ≥ 20 mg/dL, R = respiratory rate ≥ 30 breaths/minute; B = blood pressure [low systolic < 90 or diastolic ≤ 60 mmHg]; A = age ≥ 65] — Score of 3 or > predicts higher mortality.

[a] Isolation of MRSA or Pseudomonas from previous respiratory cultures in last year, hospitalization in last 90 days with IV antibiotics, or other locally validated risk factors are risks for MRSA & Pseudomonas.

[b] Consider for patients with severe inpatient CAP or in whom empiric therapy for MRSA or Pseudomonas has been started.

Treatment of Community-Acquired Pneumonia (CAP)

Setting/Situation	Treatment (Drug/Duration)
Level 1: Ambulatory Care (Empiric Options)—PSI scores of I to II and CURB-65 scores of 0 (or CURB-65 score of 1 if age > 65)	
Previously healthy and no risk factors for drug-resistant *S. pneumoniae* (DRSP) infection	• Doxycycline for 5 days[a] • Macrolide (clarithromycin; azithromycin; erythromycin) for 5 days[a]
With comorbidity (chronic heart, lung, or liver disease; diabetes; alcoholism; immunosuppression; malignancies, asplenia, or other risks for drug resistant *S. pneumoniae* infection or recent antibiotic therapy (within past 3 months)	• Fluoroquinolone (moxifloxacin, gemifloxacin, or levofloxacin 750mg) • β-lactam & Macrolide: high-dose amoxicillin (1 g three times daily) or amoxicillin clavulanate (2 g two times daily) preferred; alternatives = ceftriaxone; cefuroxime, & doxycycline
Hospitalized Patient (Empiric/Nonintensive Care Unit)—Patients SpO2 <92% on room air with significant change from baseline OR with PSI scores of ≥ III & CURB-65 scores ≥ 1 (or CURB-65 score ≥2 if age > 65)	
Patients without Methicillin-Resistant *S. aureus* (MRSA) or risk factors for pseudomonas	• Combo therapy with a β-lactam (e.g., ceftriaxone, cefotaxime, or cefpodoxime [500 mg 2 times daily]) plus either macrolide or doxycycline OR • Monotherapy with respiratory fluoroquinolone • Duration of 5 days superscript a
Patients with risk factors for pseudomonas	• Antipseudomonal β-lactam (e.g., piperacillin-tazobactam, or cefepime) + antipseudomonal fluoroquinolone (e.g., ciprofloxacin or levofloxacin 750 mg) OR • β-lactam + aminoglycoside & azithromycin OR • β-lactam + aminoglycoside & fluoroquinolone
Patients with risk factors for MRSA	• Add an agent with anti-MRSA activity: vancomycin (trough = 15 to 20 ug/mL or 15 mg/kg) or linezolid
Pathogen Specific Treatment Options	
S. pneumoniae	• Amoxicillin; ceftriaxone; cefotaxime; macrolide; fluoroquinolone
MSSA	• Cefazolin, oxacillin, nafcillin
Mycoplasma or chlamydia	• Macrolide or doxycycline for 7 days
H. influenzae	• Doxycycline; 2nd or 3rd generation cephalosporin or fluroquinolone x 1 to 2 weeks

Notes: [a]Patients with CAP should be treated for a min of 5 days, should be afebrile for 48 to 72 h, and should have no >1 CAP-associated sign of clinical instability. If clinical stability criteria (resolution of vital sign abnormalities); MSSA = Methicillin-sensitive *S. Aureus*. Additional management strategies for ICU patients not listed on this card.

Sample references: Metlay JP, Waterer GW, Long AC, et al. *Diagnosis and Treatment of Adults with Community-acquired Pneumonia. An Official Clinical Practice Guideline of the American Thoracic Society and Infectious Diseases Society of America.* Am J Respir Crit Care Med. 2019;200(7):e45-e67.

Hospital-Acquired Pneumonia (HAP) Management

Common Pathogens

- ☐ **S. aureus**
  - ☐ Methicillin-resistant S. aureus (MRSA)
  - ☐ Methicillin-sensitive S. aureus (MSSA)
- ☐ **Gram-negative bacilli**
  - ☐ Klebsiella
  - ☐ Pseudomonas aeruginosa
  - ☐ Enterobacter
  - ☐ S. maltophilia
  - ☐ E. coli
  - ☐ Acinetobacter spp.
- ☐ Legionella spp.
- ☐ **Viruses**
  - ☐ Influenza
  - ☐ RSV
  - ☐ Parainfluenza
- ☐ **Anaerobes**

Notes: Most common are MRSA and gram-negative bacilli. Most difficult to treat are P. aeruginosa & Acinetobacter.

Empiric Treatment

Based on patient's risk of multidrug resistance (MDR):
- ☐ Receipt of intravenous antibiotics during prior 90 days
- ☐ High risk of mortality

Additional risk factors for Pseudomonas

- ☐ Hospitalization in unit where > 10% of gram-negative isolates are resistant to an agent being considered for monotherapy
- ☐ Patient in septic shock
- ☐ Patient with structural lung disease (bronchiectasis; cystic fibrosis)

Additional risk factors for MRSA

- ☐ Hospitalization in unit where > 20% of S. aureus isolates are methicillin resistant
- ☐ Prevalence of MRSA unknown

Note: Refer to your institution's local susceptibilities for further guidance on empiric treatment.

Reference: Chart based on Tables 4 & 5 of ATS/IDSA Guidelines

Empiric Therapy

NOT AT HIGH RISK of Mortality & NO FACTORS Increasing Likelihood of Multidrug Resistant (MDR) Pathogens (CHOOSE ONE)

Medication	Dose[a]
Piperacillin/tazobactam[b]	4.5 g IV q6h
Cefepime[b]	2 g IV q8h
Levofloxacin	750 mg IV daily
Imipenem[b]	500 mg IV q6h
Meropenem[b]	2 grams IV q8h

CHOOSE TWO for MDR &/or Pseudomonas Risk (CHOOSE ONE β-lactam/Carbapenem & ONE from Another Class)

Medication	Dose[a]
Piperacillin/tazobactam[b]	4.5 g IV q6h
Cefepime[b]	2 g IV q8h
Ceftazidime	2 g IV q8h
Levofloxacin	750 mg IV daily
Ciprofloxacin	400 mg IV q8h
Imipenem[b]	500 mg IV q6h
Meropenem[b]	2 grams IV q8h
Amikacin	20 mg/kg IV daily
Gentamicin	7 mg/kg IV daily
Tobramycin	7 mg/kg IV daily
Aztreonam[d]	2 g IV q8h

Add for MDR and/or MRSA Risk (CHOOSE ONE)

Vancomycin[c]	15 mg/kg IV q8 to 12h Achieve trough of 15 to 20 mg/mL (consider loading dose of 25 to 30 mg/kg IV x 1 for severe illness)
Linezolid	600 mg IV q12h

[a] Alternate dosing regimens using pharmacokinetic/pharmacodynamic (PK/PD) data may be used.
[b] Extended infusions may be appropriate.
[c] Area under the curve (AUC) targets of 400 to 600 mg hr/L may be used instead of trough goals
[d] Aztreonam should only be used in patients with confirmed penicillin & cephalosporin allergy.

References: Chart based on Table 4 of 2016 IDSA HAP/VAP Guidelines. Tamma PD, Aitken SL, Bonomo RA, Mathers AJ, van Duin D, Clancy CJ. Infectious diseases society of america guidance on the treatment of extended-spectrum β-lactamase producing enterobacterales (Esbl-e), carbapenem-resistant enterobacterales (Cre), and pseudomonas aeruginosa with difficult-to-treat resistance (DTR-P. aeruginosa). Clin Infect Dis. 2021;72(7):e169[ndash]e183.

Hospital-Acquired Pneumonia (HAP) Management *(continued)*

Risk Reduction
- Effective infection control measures (education; compliance; isolation)
- Surveillance of infections to identify, quantify, & prepare
- Intubation/mechanical ventilation avoidance and duration reduction when possible (guidance exists on preferred type of intubation & tubes)
- Patient positioning (semirecumbent positioning)
- Modulation of oropharyngeal colonization by combinations of antibiotics (oral) with or without systemic therapy or selective decontamination of digestive tract (SDD)
- Consideration of risk associated with stress ulcer prophylaxis regimen or chronic proton pump inhibitor therapy
- Consideration of type of transfusion (undetermined)
- Blood glucose management

References
- Institution Specific Formulary http://www.hopkinsguides.com/hopkins/ub
- Kalil AC, Metersky ML, Klompas M, Muscedere J, Sweeney DA, et al. Management of Adults with Hospital-acquired and Ventilator-associated Pneumonia: 2016 Clinical Practice Guidelines by the Infectious Diseases Society of America and the American Thoracic Society. *Clinical Infectious Diseases* 2016; 63(5):e61–111. cid.oxfordjournals.org/content/early/2016/07/06/cid.ciw353.

Prepared by Jeanine P. Abrons, Ben Lomaestro, and Bryan P. White
Additional card updates with Adrienne Rouiller and Bryan P. White

HAP or VAP Suspected

Obtain lower respiratory tract (LRT) sample for culture & microscopy[a]

Unless there is both a low clinical suspicion for pneumonia and negative microscopy of LRT sample, begin empiric antimicrobial therapy using guideline algorithm & local microbiologic data.

Days 2 and 3:
Check cultures: assess clinical response (e.g., temperature, white blood cell, chest x-ray, purulent sputum).

Clinical improvement in 48 to 72 hours

NO

Culture –	Culture +
Search for other pathogens, complications, diagnoses, or sites of infection	Adjust antibiotic therapy; search for other pathogens, complications, diagnoses, or other sites of infection

YES

Culture –	Culture +
Consider stopping antibiotics	De-escalate antibiotics (when possible). Consider treating for 7 to 8 days; then reassess.

Suggested treatment duration of 7 days

Reference: Based on Figure 1 of ATS/IDSA Guidelines

Note: VAP = ventilator-associated pneumonia.
[a] If delays or difficulties in obtaining cultures, consider a methicillin resistant staph aureus (MRSA) polymerase chain reaction (PCR) with nasal swab to help de-escalate vancomycin.

Aminoglycosides: Traditional Considerations and Dosing in Adults

General Information

- Fight bacteria by interrupting bacterial protein synthesis.
- Bactericidal against gram-negative aerobic organisms including *Pseudomonas*
- Active against *Staphylococci* but inactive against *Streptococci*
- Synergistic with some penicillins (including ampicillin) & vancomycin against *Enterococci*
- Demonstrate concentration-dependent killing
- Have a significant postantibiotic effect
- Amount in the tissue accumulates over time contributing to toxicity
- Average volume of distribution in otherwise healthy adults = 0.26 L/kg (range 0.2 to 0.3)
- Does not distribute to adipose tissue; obese patients require a correction in weight used for V_d (patients with cystic fibrosis, ascites, or critical illness also may require corrections)
- Important adverse effects: nephrotoxicity; ototoxicity; neuromuscular blockage; rash
- Elimination closely correlated with creatinine clearance

Aminoglycoside Area	Notes/Discussion
Target Therapeutic Levels (Peaks)	• Gentamicin/tobramycin: 4 to 8 mcg/mL (normal); urinary tract infection: 4 to 5 mcg/mL; endocarditis: 3 to 4 mcg/mL; cystic fibrosis: 8 to 10 mcg/mL • Amikacin: 20 to 25 mcg/mL (traditional dosing); 40 to 100 mcg/mL (single daily dose)
Initial or Maintenance Dose	• Doses of aminoglycosides must be individualized based on the patient characteristics such as age, weight, renal function, & infection treated. ○ See side 2 of card for single daily dosing strategy; single daily dosing shown to have lower incidence & longer time to onset of nephrotoxicity than traditional dosing. • Gentamicin traditional dosing of adults (not single daily dosing) is 3 to 5 mg/kg IV or IM divided every 8 hours until over the age of 60 (then, 3 mg/kg divided every 12 hours) • Tobramycin traditional dosing of adults: 1 to 2 mg/kg IV over 30 minutes every 8 hours • Amikacin traditional dosing of adults: 5 mg/kg IV over 30 min every 8 hours or 7.5 mg/kg over 30 min every 12 hours • Dose adjustments must be made based on renal function. • Other certain populations also require dosage adjustments (e.g., based on postmenstrual age (gentamicin), for cystic fibrosis, for hemodialysis (postdialysis dosing)) • This dosing reflects adult dosing & not dosing used on neonatal or pediatric patient population.
Other Monitoring (Beyond peak and trough levels)	**Monitoring Parameter** Blood urea nitrogen (BUN) — Weight Serum creatinine — Hearing
Recommendations for Monitoring Levels	• Ensure proper timing of sampling to enable accurate interpretation of levels. Note time samples were drawn & when infusions were started/stopped. • Sampling for peak in traditional dosing completed 20 to 30 minutes following infusion; 1 hour for single daily dosing.

Commonly Used Abbreviations

Term	Definition	Term	Definition
TBW	total body weight	CrCl	creatinine clearance in mL/min
IBW	ideal body weight	SCr	serum creatinine
NS	normal saline		

Prepared by Ben Lomaestro and Bryan P. White; updated by Bryan P. White

Aminoglycosides: Single Daily Dosing

Step	Description
1) Initial Aminoglycoside Dose Given as a Single Daily Dose (SDD)	Suggested initial dosing:

Drug	DOSE — Normal	DOSE — Critically Ill/Septic Patient
Gentamicin	6 mg/kg	7 mg/kg
Tobramycin	6 mg/kg	7 mg/kg
Amikacin	24 mg/kg	30 to 40 mg/kg

Use TBW unless patient weight is > 40% above the IBW; then consider use of adjusted body weight or ideal body weight.

2) Determination of Dosing Interval

- Dosing interval is based upon estimated CrCl.

$$CrCl = \frac{(140 - age) \times IBW \text{ (in kg)} \times (0.85 \text{ in females})}{(72 \times SCr)}$$

- Determine the initial dosing interval

Calculated CrCl	Initial Dosing Interval
60 mL/min or >	Every 24 hours
40 to 60 mL/min	x1 dose based on drug levels

3) Administration

- Administration time over 1 hour or consult institution specific guidelines.
- Following infusion with a flush of 50 mL NS to ensure dose administered.
- Record actual start & stop time.

4) Serum Concentration Monitoring

- Obtain PEAK concentration 1 hour after END of infusion.
- Obtain a second or RANDOM concentration between 8 & 10 hours after END of infusion.
- Record ACTUAL time sampled.
- Record ACTUAL start and stop time of infusion & state "single dose interval."
- Trough levels should be undetectable with SDD.

5) Dosage/Regimen Adjustment Based on Table

- Adjust dosage regimen based on serum concentrations. Dosage changes result in proportional changes in serum concentrations.

PEAK (1 hour post infusion) concentration interpretation (use higher level for resistant organisms)

Drug	Recommended Action Based on PEAK Concentration	
Gentamicin and Tobramycin	**Concentration**	**Course of Action**
	7 mg/kg levels also can be evaluated based on the Hartford nomogram	
	> 25 mcg/mL	Reduce dose to achieve peak < 25 mcg/mL
	10 to 25 mcg/mL	Maintain dose
	< 10 mcg/mL	Increase dose to achieve level > 10 mcg/mL
Amikacin	**Concentration**	**Course of Action**
	> 100 mcg/mL	Reduce dose to achieve first level < 100 mcg/mL
	40 to 100 mcg/mL	Maintain dose
	< 40 mcg/mL	Increase dose to achieve level > 40 mcg/mL

Reference: Nicolau DP, Freeman CD, Belliveau PP, Nightingale CH, Ross JW, Quintiliani R. Experience with a once-daily aminoglycoside program administered to 2,184 adult patients. Antimicrob Agents Chemother. 1995;39(3):650–5.

Note: Use institution-specific dosing guidelines if available. For abbreviations, see previous page.

Prepared by Ben Lomaestro and Bryan P. White; updated by Bryan P. White

Vancomycin: Considerations and Dosing in Adults

Dosing Consideration	Notes/Discussion
Pharmacokinetic Exposure Target	• Other indications: 10 to 15 mcg/mL • Bacteremia, meningitis, osteomyelitis, pneumonia, endocarditis, and necrotizing fasciitis: AUC of 400 to 600[a]
Initial or Maintenance Dose (For *C. difficile* colitis dosing—See side 2 of card) *= Administer longer than 1 hour for doses > 1 g	• Typical dosing is based upon actual body weight. • In morbidly obese adults: Use of AUC monitoring and population equations is recommended. Initial doses often don't exceed 4500 mg.

Population	Dosing Based on Trough
Individuals < 65 Years of Age	• **Trough Targets of 10 to 15 mcg/mL**: 15 mg/kg or 1 g intravenous (IV) every 8 to 12 hours over at least 1 hour*. Frequency based on renal function (see below).
Individuals > 65 Years of Age	• **Trough Targets of 10 to 15 mcg/mL**: 15 mg/kg or 1 g IV over at least 1 hour.* No more often than every 12 hours initially—if CrCl < 50 mL/min give every 24 hours; If CrCl < 20 mL/min, give initial dose and base subsequent doses on drug levels.
AUC dosing	• Consider loading with 25 to 30 mg/kg (max 3 grams) IV at a rate of 1 g/hour[b,c]

Dose Adjustments Made Based on Renal Impairment		
> 90	15 mg/kg to 20 mg/kg every 12 hours	Every 24 to 48 hours (monitor levels)
51 to 89	10 to 15 mg/kg every 24 hours	750 mg to 1 g ONCE (monitor levels)
30 to 50	10 to 15 mg/kg every 24 hours	Based on levels and targeting trough—see reference for more information
20 to 29	5 to 10 mg/kg every 24 hours	
Hemodialysis		
CRRT	Single initial dose based on target and weight as above with monitoring of random levels	

Adverse Effects	• Rapid infusions may produce flushing or rash (vancomycin infusion reaction) possibly accompanied by hypotension due to release of histamine. Slow infusions over 1 hour to reduce risk. Local reactions at site of administration; nephrotoxicity; ototoxicity; leukopenia; eosinophilia; thrombocytopenia; chills; nausea; fever muscle aches; autoimmune reactions

Notes on Use and Interpretation:
- Always refer to local institutional practices/recommendations of antimicrobial stewardship when available.
- For larger infusions, administer no faster than 1 g/hour to reduce risk of vancomycin infusion reaction.
- Variations in dosing may exist dependent on institution.

Prepared by Ben Lomaestro and Bryan P. White

Sampling Time
Trough: 1 hour or less before next dose; generally draw 1st trough prior to 3rd or 4th dose; vancomycin level(s) for AUC calculations should be drawn at steady with peaks 1 to 2 hours after end of infusion & troughs 30 minutes before the dose for the trapezoidal method.

References
Crew P, Heintz SJ, Heintz BH. Vancomycin dosing and monitoring for patients with end-stage renal disease receiving intermittent hemodialysis. *Am J Health Syst Pharm.* 2015;72(21):1856–64.

Note: [a]Use of AUC vs trough in CNS infections is debated in the literature. AUC of 400 to 600 assumes a vancomycin minimum inhibitory concentration (MIC) = 1 in methicillin-resistant staph aureus (MRSA). For patients with MICs to vancomycin > 1, alternative therapies should be considered; [b]Recommendations based on the Matzke equation & may not be accurate in obese or critically ill patients. Consider using a local calculator or Bayesian program for these patients if available. [c]Patients in acute kidney injury, on renal replacement therapy, or with creatinine clearances < 20 mL/minute should initially be dosed with 15 to 20 mg/kg (max 2 grams) with random levels instead of AUC dosing.

References: Rybak MJ, Le J, Lodise TP, et al. Therapeutic monitoring of vancomycin for serious methicillin-resistant Staphylococcus aureus infections: A revised consensus guideline and review by the American Society of Health-System Pharmacists, the Infectious Diseases Society of America, the Pediatric Infectious Diseases Society, and the Society of Infectious Diseases Pharmacists. *Am J Health Syst Pharm.* 2020;77(11):835–64. Crass RL, Dunn R, Hong J, Krop LC, Pai MP. Dosing vancomycin in the super obese: less is more. *J Antimicrob Chemother.* 2018;73(11):3081–3086

Vancomycin: General Information and Dosing (PO/IV) for *C. difficile* Colitis

General Information:

Vancomycin
- Glycopeptide antimicrobial effective against gram-positive organisms including *Streptococci*, *Staphylococci* (including methicillin-resistant *Staphylococcus aureus* [MRSA]), & coagulase-negative *Staphylococci*.
- Bacteriostatic against *Enterococci*; bactericidal against *Corynebacterium* and *Clostridia*.
- Use by mouth or per rectum for *C. difficile colitis*.
- Pregnancy category: C
- Lactation: Considered safe
- Critical drug interactions: Use caution in combining IV vancomycin with nephrotoxic or ototoxic agents such as aminoglycosides piperacillin/tazobactam, amphotericin B & cisplatin; cholestyramine & colestipol bind to vancomycin & are contraindicated when using vancomycin for *C. difficile colitis*.

C. difficile Colitis Category	Corresponding Vancomycin Dosing (From IDSA Guidelines)
Initial Episode, Mild to Severe	• Vancomycin 125 mg by mouth every 6 hours for 10 days. • Metronidazole 500 mg every 8 hours for 10 days may be used if oral vancomycin & fidaxomicin are not available.[a] • Fidaxomicin 200 mg PO twice daily for 10 days.
Initial Episode, Fulminant/ICU	• 500 mg every 6 hours (4 times per day) by mouth or nasogastric tube plus metronidazole 500 mg every 8 hours IV. If complete ileus, consider adding rectal installation of vancomycin.
Initial/First Recurrence	• Use vancomycin taper regimen: 125 mg 4 times per day for 10 to 14 days 2 times per week for 1 week, 1 time per day for 1 week, then every 2 or 4 days for 2 to 8 weeks.
Severe/Complicated or ICU	• 500 mg by mouth every 6 hours plus metronidazole 500 mg IV every 8 hours & if patient has ileus rectal vancomycin • Fidaxomicin 10 day course or extended pulse (bid for 5 days, then every 48 hours from days 7–25)
Recurrent (Second and Greater)	• Fidaxomicin 200 mg PO twice daily for 10 days should be considered for 2nd recurrence if a patient has failed vancomycin & vancomycin taper. Fecal microbiota transplantation should be considered for the 3rd recurrence. • Fidaxomicin extended pulse (bid for 5 days, then every 48 hours from days 7–25) is also an option.
Clinical Definition	**Supportive Clinical Data from *C. difficile* Guidelines**
Initial Episode; Mild to Moderate	• Leukocytosis with white blood cells (WBC) of 15,000 cells/µL or **lower** & SCr level <1.5 times premorbid level
Initial Episode; Severe	• Leukocytosis with WBCs of 15,000 cells/µL or higher & SCr ≥ 1.5 times premorbid level
Initial Episode; Severe Complicated	• Hypotension or shock, ileus, or megacolon

Notes: [a]The IDSA guidelines prefer fidaxomicin first line over vancomycin. The ACG guidelines don't have a preference.
Bezlotoxumab may be considered for patients at high risk of recurrence.

Recommended Resources/References
- Kullar R, Leonard SN, Davis SL, Delgado G, Pogue JM et al. Validation of the effectiveness of vancomycin nomogram in achieving target trough concentrations of 15 to 20 mg/L Suggested by the Vancomycin Consensus Guidelines. *Pharmacotherapy*. 2011. 31(5): 441–48.
- Johnson S, Lavergne V, Skinner AM, et al. Clinical practice guideline by the infectious diseases society of america (Idsa) and society for healthcare epidemiology of america (Shea) 2021 focused update guidelines on management of clostridioides difficile infection in adults. *Clinical Infectious Diseases*. 2021;73(5):e1029–e1044.
- Kelly CR, Fischer M, Allegretti JR, et al. Acg clinical guidelines: prevention, diagnosis, and treatment of clostridioides difficile infections. *Am J Gastroenterol*. 2021;116(6):1124–1147.

Prepared by Ben Lomaestro and Bryan P. White; updated by Bryan P. White

Sample Antimicrobial Coverage

Penicillins

Penicillin Antibiotic	Gram (+)	Enterococcus*	MSSA**	MRSA	Gram (−)	Pseudomonas	Anaerobes	Atypicals
Penicillin G	+++	++/+	−	−	−	−	−	−
Penicillin V	+++	++/+	−	−	−	−	−	−
Ampicillin	+++	++/+	−	−	+/++	−	−	−
Amoxicillin	+++	++/+	−	−	+/++	−	−	−
Oxacillin	+++	−	+++	−	−	−	−	−
Dicloxacillin	+++	−	+++	−	−	−	−	−
Amoxicillin/Clavulanate	+++	++/+	+++	−	+/++	−	+++	−
Ampicillin/Sulbactam	+++	++/+	+++	−	+/++	−	+++	−
Piperacillin/Tazobactam	+++	++/+	++	−	+++	+++	+++	−

MSSA = methicillin sensitive staph aureus; MRSA = methicillin resistant staph aureus

Key: − = no coverage; + = weak coverage; ++ = moderate coverage

Notes: *Enterococcus coverage represents enterococcus faecalis; only ~ 10 to 20% of enterococcus faecium are susceptible. **Over ~90% of MSSA have penicillinases that will break down penicillin & amoxicillin.

Prepared by Bryan White and Jeanine Abrons

Sample Antimicrobial Coverage *(continued)*

Cephalosporins, Carbapenems, & Monobactams

Cephalosporin Antibiotic	Gram (+)	Enterococcus	MSSA	MRSA	Gram (−)	Pseudomonas	Anaerobes	Atypicals
Cefazolin	+++	−	+++	−	+	−	−	−
Cephalexin	+++	−	+++	−	+	−	−	−
Cefuroxime	+++	−	+++	−	++	−	−	−
Ceftriaxone	+++	−	+/++	−	++/++[#]	−	−	−
Cefepime	+++	−	++	−	+++	+++	−	−

[#]*Note: Does not cover extended spectrum beta-lactamase producing Enterobacteriaceae (ESBLs), which are more common in inpatient settings.*

MSSA = methicillin sensitive staph aureus; MRSA = methicillin resistant staph aureus

Key: − = no coverage; + = weak coverage; ++ = moderate coverage; +++ = strong coverage

Carbapenem Antibiotic	Gram (+)	Enterococcus[†]	MSSA	MRSA	Gram (−)	Pseudomonas	Anaerobes	Atypicals
Meropenem	+++	++	+++	−	+++	+++	+++	−
Ertapenem	+++	−	+++	−	+++	−	+++	−
Imipenem & Cilastin	+++	++	+++	−	+++	+++	+++	−
Doripenem	+++	++	+++	−	+++	+++	+++	−

[†]*Note: Enterococcus coverage represents enterococcus faecalis; only ~ 10 to 20% of enterococcus faecium are susceptible.*

Monobactam Antibiotic	Gram (+)	Enterococcus	MSSA	MRSA	Gram (−)	Pseudomonas	Anaerobes	Atypicals
Azteonam	−	−	−	−	++/+++	++	−	−

Prepared by Bryan White and Jeanine Abrons

Sample Antimicrobial Coverage *(continued)*

Macrolides, Quinolones, Tetracyclines, & Aminoglycosides

Macrolide Antibiotic	Gram (+)	Enterococcus	MSSA	MRSA	Gram (−)	Pseudomonas	Anaerobes	Atypicals
Erythromycin	++	−	++	−	+/++	−	−	+++
Azithromycin	+++	−	+	−	++	−	−	+++

MSSA = methicillin sensitive staph aureus; MRSA = methicillin resistant staph aureus

Key: − = no coverage; + = weak coverage; ++ = moderate coverage; +++ = strong coverage

Quinolone Antibiotic	Gram (+)	Enterococcus	MSSA	MRSA	Gram (−)	Pseudomonas	Anaerobes	Atypicals
Ciprofloxacin	+/++	+	++	−	++/+	+++	−	+++
Levofloxacin	+++	+/++	+++	−	++/+[a]	++/+++	−	+++
Moxifloxacin	+++	+/++	+++	−	++	−	++	+++

[a]: 20% resistance to E.coli in most centers.

Tetracycline Antibiotic	Gram (+)	Enterococcus	MSSA	MRSA	Gram (−)	Pseudomonas	Anaerobes	Atypicals
Doxycycline	++	−	++	++	++	−	−	+++
Minocycline	++	−	++	++	++	−	−	+++
Tigecycline	+++	+++	+++	+++	++	−	+++	+++

Aminoglycoside Antibiotic	Gram (+)	Enterococcus	MSSA	MRSA	Gram (−)	Pseudomonas	Anaerobes	Atypicals
Gentamicin	++	++	++	+++	+++	++	−	−
Tobramycin	−	+/++	+/++	+/++	+++	+++	−	−
Amikacin	−	−	−	−	+++	+++	−	−

Sample Antimicrobial Coverage *(continued)*

Glycopeptides & Other Antibiotics

Glycopeptide & Other Antibiotics	Gram (+)	Enterococcus	MSSA	MRSA	Gram (–)	Pseudomonas	Anaerobes	Atypicals
Vancomycin (Glycopeptide)	+++	+++	++	+++	–	–	–	–
Dalbavancin	+++	+/+	+++	+++	–	–	–	–
Oritavancin	+++	+++	+++	+++	=	=	=	=
Telavancin	+++	+++	+++	+++	–	–	–	–

MSSA – = methicillin sensitive staph aureus; MRSA = methicillin resistant staph aureus

Key — – = no coverage; +/++ = weak to moderate coverage; +++ = strong coverage

Antibiotic (Antibiotic Type)	Gram (+)	Enterococcus	MSSA	MRSA	Gram (–)	Pseudomonas	Anaerobes	Atypicals
Sulfamethoxazole/Trimethoprime (Sulfonamides)	+/++	–	++	++	++/++	–	–	–
Clindamycin (Linomycin)	+++	–	+++	+/++	–	–	+/++[#]	–
Metronidazole (Nitroimidazoles)	–	–	–	–	–	–	+++	–
Linezolid (Oxazolidinone)	+++	+++	+++	+++	–	–	–	–
Daptomycin (Cyclic Lipopeptide)	+++	+++	+++	+++	–	–	+/++[##]	–
Tigecycline (Glycylcycline)	+++	+++	+++	+++	+++	–	+++	+++

[#]: *Clindamycin does not cover gram negative anaerobes.* [##]: *Some gram positive anaerobic coverage present.*

Prepared by Bryan White and Jeanine Abrons

Gram Stain Interpretation: GRAM + RESULT

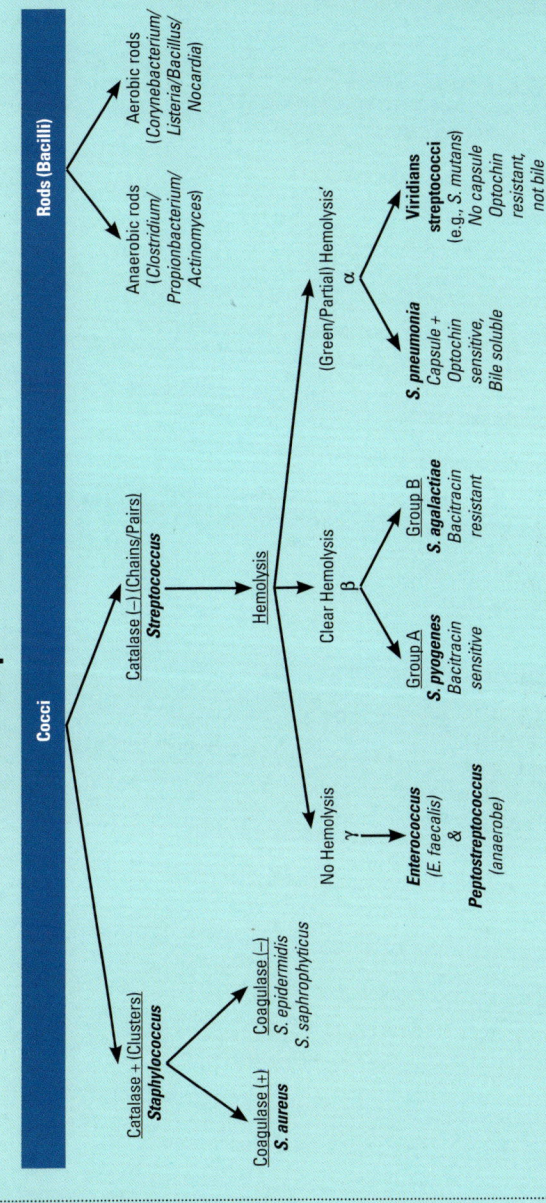

Cocci

Catalase + (Clusters) — **Staphylococcus**
- Coagulase (+) **S. aureus**
- Coagulase (−): S. epidermidis, S. saphrophyticus

Catalase (−) (Chains/Pairs) — **Streptococcus**

No Hemolysis (γ) → **Enterococcus** (E. faecalis) & **Peptostreptococcus** (anaerobe)

Hemolysis
- **Clear Hemolysis (β)**
  - Group A — **S. pyogenes** — Bacitracin sensitive
  - Group B — **S. agalactiae** — Bacitracin resistant
- **(Green/Partial) Hemolysis (α)**
  - **S. pneumonia** — Capsule +, Optochin sensitive, Bile soluble
  - **Viridians streptococci** (e.g., S. mutans) — No capsule, Optochin resistant, not bile

Rods (Bacilli)
- Anaerobic rods (Clostridium/Propionbacterium/Actinomyces)
- Aerobic rods (Corynebacterium/Listeria/Bacillus/Nocardia)

Modified based on:
Giuliano C, Patel CR, Kale-Pradhan PB. A Guide to Bacterial Culture Identification and Results Interpretation. 2019 Apr. 44(4):192–200.
Gomella LG, Haist ST: Clinician's Pocket Reference, 11th Edition; Nebraska Medicine. Antimicrobial & Clinical Microbiology Guidebook. Available at: https://www.unmc.edu/intmed/divisions/id/asp/ID_guidebook.pdf. Accessed November 2021.

Gram Stain Interpretation: GRAM – RESULT

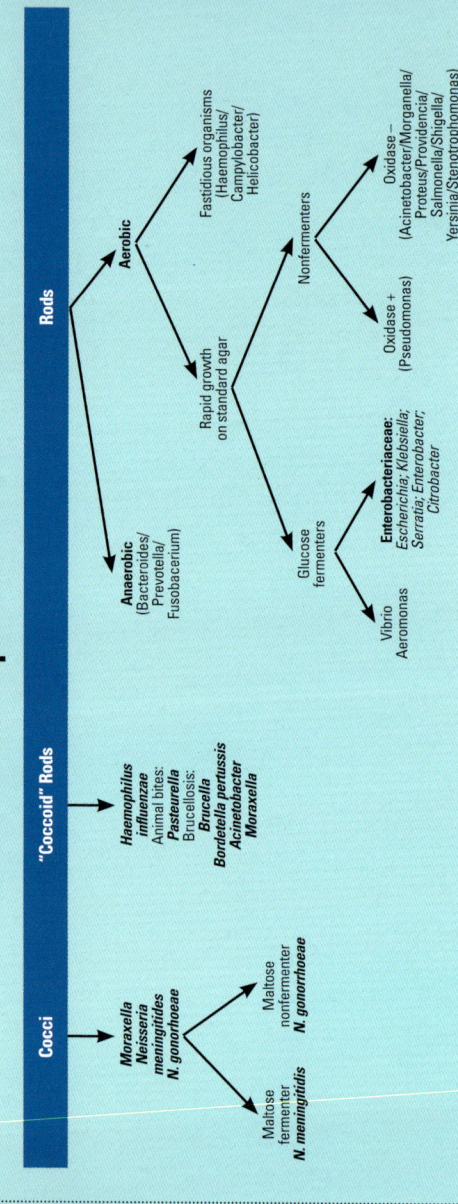

Cocci

Moraxella
Neisseria meningitidis
N. gonorrhoeae

- Maltose fermenter → *N. meningitidis*
- Maltose nonfermenter → *N. gonorrhoeae*

"Coccoid" Rods

Haemophilus influenzae
Animal bites: **Pasteurella**
Brucellosis: **Brucella**
Bordetella pertussis
Acinetobacter
Moraxella

Rods

Anaerobic
(Bacteroides/Prevotella/Fusobacterium)

Aerobic

- **Fastidious organisms** (Haemophilus/Campylobacter/Helicobacter)
- **Rapid growth on standard agar**
  - **Glucose fermenters**
    - Vibrio, Aeromonas
    - **Enterobacteriaceae:** *Escherichia; Klebsiella; Serratia; Enterobacter; Citrobacter*
  - **Nonfermenters**
    - Oxidase + (Pseudomonas)
    - Oxidase – (Acinetobacter/Morganella/Proteus/Providencia/Salmonella/Shigella/Yersinia/Stenotrophomonas)

How to Read Cultures/Sensitivities:
1) Read the source (blood, sputum, etc.).
2) Determine the status of the gram stain (preliminary vs. final). This will tell you general information that you can use to determine possible causative organisms (see Gram Stain Interpretation Charts).
3) Look at the Minimum Inhibitory Concentration (MIC) - this is listed beside a drug & represents the lowest concentration of the drug that will prevent visible growth of the bacteria. Note: the lowest MIC does not always indicate the best activity. You must compare the MIC listed to the specific breakpoint for that bug/drug pair. Breakpoints can be found on the Clinical & Laboratory Standards Institute (CLSI) website. They publish yearly the M100 *Performance Standards for Antimicrobial Susceptibility Testing*. The newest version is the CLSI M100-ED31:2021 and can be found at http://em100.edaptivedocs.net/GetDoc.aspx?doc=CLSI%20M100%20ED31:2021&scope=user.
4) Read the interpretation column: S = Susceptible; I = Intermittent; R = Resistant

Other Notes on Gram Stain Interpretation
Note: Some institutions no longer report B-hemolytic strep in cultures. This is sometimes reported or identified using rapid diagnostic tools in an outpatient/inpatient setting.

Modified based on:
Gomella LG, Haist ST: Clinician's Pocket Reference, 11th Edition & Guzman OE. Chapter 32 – Antibiotic Streamlining. Competence Assessment Tools for Health-System Pharmacies. Available at: https://www.ashp.org/-/media/store-files/p4023-sample-chapter-32.ashx. Nebraska Medicine Antimicrobial Guide: https://www.unmc.edu/intmed/divisions/id/asp/ID_guidebook.pdf (Accessed November 2021) & Gallagher JC, MacDougall C. Antibiotics Simplified – 3rd edition © Jones & Bartlett Publishing

Consideration of When to Draw Cultures and Start Antibiotics in the Emergency Department (ED)

Shapiro Criteria

One of the following
- Temp > 39.4 C (103 F)
- Suspected endocarditis
- Indwelling vascular catheter

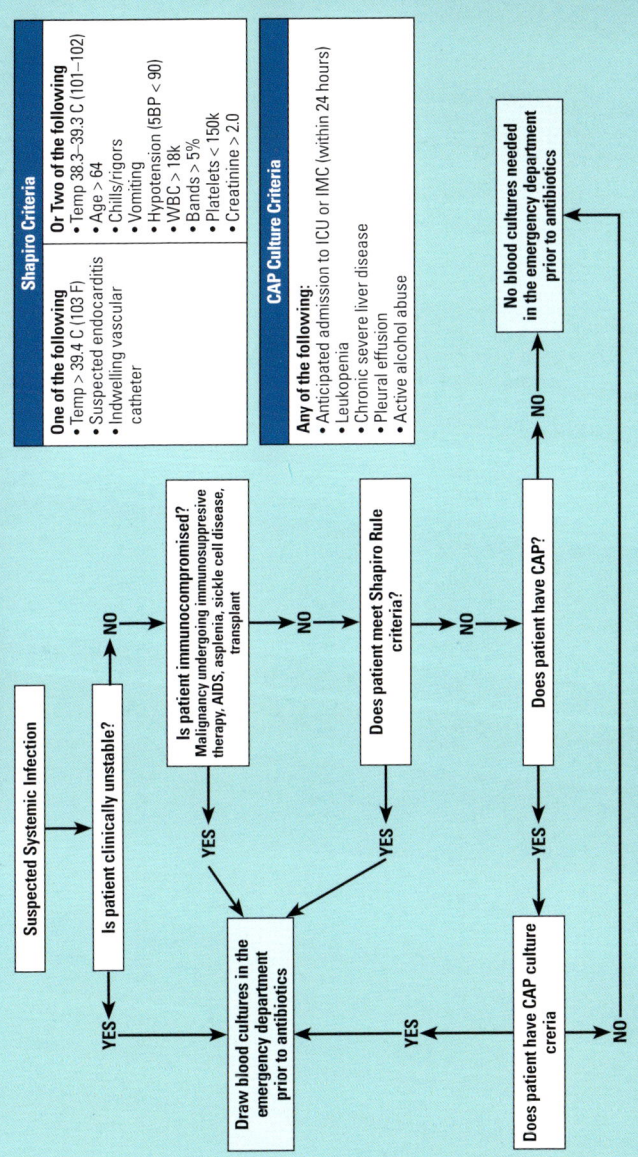

Or Two of the following
- Temp 38.3–39.3 C (101–102)
- Age > 64
- Chills/rigors
- Vomiting
- Hypotension (SBP < 90)
- WBC > 18k
- Bands > 5%
- Platelets < 150k
- Creatinine > 2.0

CAP Culture Criteria

Any of the following:
- Anticipated admission to ICU or IMC (within 24 hours)
- Leukopenia
- Chronic severe liver disease
- Pleural effusion
- Active alcohol abuse

Suspected Systemic Infection

→ Is patient clinically unstable?
- YES → Draw blood cultures in the emergency department prior to antibiotics
- NO → Is patient immunocompromised? (Malignancy undergoing immunosuppresive therapy, AIDS, asplenia, sickle cell disease, transplant)
  - YES → Draw blood cultures in the emergency department prior to antibiotics
  - NO → Does patient meet Shapiro Rule criteria?
    - YES → Draw blood cultures in the emergency department prior to antibiotics
    - NO → Does patient have CAP?
      - YES → Does patient have CAP culture criteria?
        - YES → Draw blood cultures in the emergency department prior to antibiotics
        - NO → No blood cultures needed in the emergency department prior to antibiotics
      - NO → No blood cultures needed in the emergency department prior to antibiotics

---

CAP = community acquired pneumonia; SBP = systolic blood pressure; WBC = white blood cells

Based on Pawlowicz A, Holland C, Zou B, Payton T, Tyndall JA, Allen B. Implementation of an evidence-based algorithm reduces blood culture overuse in an adult emergency department. Gen Int Med Clin Innov, 2016. doi:10.15761/GIMCI.1000108

Guzman GE. Chapter 32 – Antibiotic Streamlining. Competence Assessment Tools for Health-System Pharmacies. Available at: https://www.ashp.org/-/media/store-files/p4023-sample-chapter-32.ashx. Accessed December 2020.

Diagnosis and Treatment of Adults with Community-acquired Pneumonia-An Official Clinical Practice Guideline of the American Thoracic Society and Infectious Diseases Society of America (https://www.atsjournals.org/doi/pdf/10.1164/rccm.201908-1581ST)

Consider When to & Whether to Draw a Culture

Number & Timing	• Perform cultures before starting antibiotics if possible • Do not delay antibiotics if life-threatening condition: start broad & de-escalate • Consider collection of 2 to 3 sets of separately collected blood cultures to detect bacteremia • When other blood work is done, collect blood culture first
Control the Source	• Consider incision/drainage, device removal, debridement, & amputation when possible

Contamination & Colonization	• Signs of Possible Contamination/Colonization: Large # of epithelial cells present/growth of normal skin flora
	• Consider: Was the specimen collected properly?
	   ○ *Meticulous skin antisepsis*
	   ○ *Site of collection*
	   ○ *Volume of sample*

Presence of Signs of Infection	• Fever >100.4 (38 degrees C):
	   ○ *Note: Not for all patients; elderly may be hypothermic*
	• Systolic blood pressure (BP) < 90 mmHg
	   ○ *Cause = dehydration/sepsis*
	• Heart rate > 100 bpm
	• Rapid breathing (> 20 bpm or PaCO2 < 32 mmHg if MV)
	• WBC > 4,000 to 12,000 cells/mm^3 with possible left shift
	• PCT > 0.5 ng/mL

Other Factors	• Previous use of current antimicrobial therapy (possible false negative)

MV = mechanical ventilation; WBC = white blood cells; PCT = procalcitonin

Note: Lamy B, Dargere S, Arendrup MC, Parienti JJ, Tattevin P. How to optimize the use of blood cultures for the diagnosis of bloodstream infections? State-of-the-art. Frontiers in Microbiology. 2016 May 12; 7: 697

Chapter 32 – Antibiotic Streamlining. Competence Assessment Tools for Health-System Pharmacies. Available at: https://www.ashp.org/-/media/store-files/p4023-sample-chapter-32

Examples of Considerations by Culture Type

Notes

Blood culture	• Make sure to properly clean puncture site of with alcohol followed by chlorhexidine • Collect 1 culture for aerobes/anaerobes & 2 or 3 cultures by separate stick per septic episode • For laboratory confirmation: 1 positive blood culture with recognized pathogen from venipuncture; for skin organisms: > 2 cultures on separate occasions positive for same organism + clinic symptoms • For suspected catheter-related bloodstream infection draw 1 set from device & 1 from separate venipuncture (must be positive with same organism with clinical signs/symptoms) • Consider differential time to positivity to confirm catheter-related bloodstream infection, defined as growth of microbes from a blood sample drawn from a catheter tip at least 2 hours before microbial growth is detected in a blood culture from a peripheral site. The thought is that the bacterial burden is higher, & it should grow the same organism.*
Wound/abscess	• Ensure wound/abscess was cleaned with 70% alcohol & allowed to dry • Pus of fluid should be aspirated if possible then transported via syringe or appropriate transport vial/tube • Discourage swabs due to insufficient material for gram stain • Obtain a deep culture or biopsy whenever possible
Urine	• Collection done via midstream with 1st portion of urine discarded • Do not treat asymptomatic bacteriuria except in pregnancy or GU instrumentation

From: https://academic.oup.com/cid/article/49/1/1/369414#210121434 (Accessed November 2021)

Initial Card by Anastasia Lundt and Jeanine P. Abrons; updated by Michael Parisi-Mercado and Jeanine P. Abrons

Information for Pharmacists for Parents During COVID-19

General Tips for Talking to Children About COVID-19	Well-Child Care and Immunizations During the COVID-19 Pandemic
• Remain calm. Remember that children react to both what you say and also how you say it; they also pick up cues in your conversations with others. • Reassure children that they will be safe. • Stress that it is OK to feel upset and share how you deal or cope with your emotions related to COVID-19. • Talk and listen. Encourage questions. • Avoid blaming others. • Monitor what children see and hear—too much information can be anxiety provoking. • Teach children general measures to reduce the spread of germs. • Encourage role-playing how to communicate with other children about COVID-19. Clarify the importance of vaccines and provide information on where vaccines are accessible.	• Children are at risk for vaccine-preventable diseases and are recommended to continue to follow the normal vaccination schedule. • Surveillance and screening of children should be continued in either in-office or telehealth visits. • Newborns should be seen within 3 to 5 days of birth after hospital discharge and ideally in-person.

Consider Techniques to Create Positive Pediatric Vaccine Experience:
- Colorful bandaids or stickers to remove the focus of the child from the syringe or vaccine.
- Partnerships with child life specialists.
- Creating info-graphics walking the child and the parent through the process prior to the vaccine appointment.
- Movies or music to avoid apprehension in listening to others experience.
- Empowering the child with choice (e.g., bandaid, position, coping options) and having the parent discuss in advance.

Resources:
- Center for Disease Control COVID-19 Parental Resource Kit. "Ensuring Children and Young People's Social, Emotional, and Mental Well-being." https://www.cdc.gov/coronavirus/2019-ncov/daily-life-coping/parental-resource-kit/index.html (Accessed November 2021)
- "Conversation Starters to Speak with Children About COVID" (refer to reference above).
- National Association of School Psychologists: https://www.nasponline.org/resources-and-publications/resources-and-podcasts/school-climate-safety-and-crisis/health-crisis-resources/helping-children-cope-with-changes-resulting-from-covid-19 (Accessed November 2021)
- American Academy of Pediatrics. "COVID-19 in Children & Masks in Children": https://www.healthychildren.org/English/Pages/default.aspx (Accessed November 2021)

Card written by Lane Nguyen, Loc Nguyen and Jeanine P. Abrons

Usual Pediatric Dosages of Common Over-the-Counter (OTC) Medications

Background/Considerations

- Over-the-counter (OTC) medications may not be labeled for use in infants or young children.
- Dosages listed represent acceptable clinical practice; dosages not listed in labeling should be given under physician guidance. Doses bolded with asterisks (*) are doses recommended for that patient group, but should be given with physician guidance.
- Weight-based dosing is preferred over age-based dosing when provided. It is important to determine an accurate weight. Always double-check dosing.
- Parents should be reminded to check expiration dates on medications at home before giving medicines to children.
- Doses may be recommended by the pharmacy, but the caregiver may not buy the medication because they have it at home. Instruct the parent or caregiver to check the medication strength to ensure that dosing & amounts are correct.

Administration Considerations

Measurement Considerations:

- Ensure the care provider has an appropriate measuring device & demonstrate how much medication to fill on the device. If a medication comes with a device, that device should be used.
- When giving a volume to the care provider to draw up, make sure to recommend a quantity that is easily measurable with the device being used, such as a dosing spoon or syringe. Marking on the syringe or drawing the syringe on paper to indicate the appropriate amount may help to ensure recall of correct volume.
  - *Per the Institute for Safe Medication Practices (ISMP) recommendations, devices should only have metric units as measurements.*
  - *Parents of infants may wish to administer doses in smaller portions of the full dose at a time. This ensures that the parent will be able to quantify the amount that has been given in the event that the child spits up a portion of the medication.*

Taste Considerations:

- If a child does not like the taste of the medication, it may be possible to help mask the flavor by adding the medication to other liquids (e.g., juices) or semisolids (e.g., pudding). Check "Administration" section of package insert or a pediatric-specific drug reference to determine what is okay and what should be avoided.
  - *Adding medications to these substances may result in the child refusing to ingest the full amount of the medication, making it difficult to quantify the dose given.*
  - *If medication is added to other substances, use a small amount of the other substance. This ensures that all of the mixture (thus, the full dose of the medication) can be administered as a small quantity. If the child wants more of the substance, additional amounts can be given without the drug.*
- If medication is given via a tube, please check with the care provider or patient to see if they can use regular oral syringes or need additional devices.

Cough/Cold/Allergy

The Food and Drug Administration (FDA) and American Academy of Pediatrics (AAP) have issued public health advisories strongly recommending that over-the-counter cough & cold products should not be used in infants and children < 2 years of age. An advisory was originally issued in 2007. In 2008, voluntary removal of OTC infant products (products targeted at children less than 2 years of age) began due to safety concerns mentioned previously.

Sample Resources

Medication Safety for Children. *Arch Pediatr Adolesc Med.* 2010;164(2):208 in JAMA Pediatrics: Advice for Patients: (http://archpedi.jamanetwork.com/article.aspx?articleid=382713).
https://www.fda.gov/forconsumers/consumerupdates/consumerupdatesenespanol/ucm291741.htm (Accessed November 2021).
Dundee FD, Dundee DM, Noday DM. Pediatric Counseling and Medication Management Services: Opportunities for Community Pharmacists. *J Am Pharm Assoc.* 2002;42:556–567.
https://www.fda.gov/drugs/resourcesforyou/ucm133419.htm (Accessed November 2021)

Prepared by Mark Botti; updated by Kelly Shea and Jeanine Abrons

Pediatric Commercially Available Dosage Forms and Doses/Concentrations of Analgesics

Acetaminophen

Weight (in pounds [lb])	Dose (in milligrams [mg])	Dose (in milliliters [mL] of 160 mg/5 mL)
6 to 11	40*	1.25*
12 to 17	80*	2.5*
18 to 23	120*	3.75*
24 to 35	160	5
36 to 47	240	7.5
48 to 59	320	10
60 to 71	400	12.5
72 to 95	480	15

Doses can be given every 4 to 6 hours. Do not give more than 5 doses in 24 hours.
Maximum daily dose is 480 mg per dose up to 5 doses, or 2400 mg total daily dose.

Liquids are available as elixir grape, cherry, berry, fruit, bubble gum, cotton candy, & strawberry. Oral disintegrating tablets are available as grape, wild grape, & bubble gum flavors. Sugar-free & gluten-free preparations exist. Preparations come in alcohol-free and dye-free varieties.

Ibuprofen

Weight (in pounds [lb])	Dose (in milligrams [mg])
Less than 12	Not recommended
12 to 17	50*
18 to 23	75*
24 to 35	100
36 to 47	150
48 to 59	200
60 to 71	250
72 to 95	300

Doses can be given every 6 to 8 hours.
Maximum daily dose is 40 mg/kg/day up to 1200 mg/day. Maximum of 4 doses per day.
Available as an oral suspension with flavors of fruit, grape, blue-raspberry, white grape, berry, tropical punch, & bubble gum. Comes in alcohol-free, dye-free, & sugar-free varieties. Chewable tabs available in grape & orange flavors.

Medication / Dosage Forms / Doses and Concentrations

Medication	Dosage Forms	Doses and Concentrations of Commercially Available Products
Acetaminophen	Chewable tablets	80 mg
	Liquid	160 mg/5 mL
	Orally disintegrating tablets	80 mg, 160 mg
	Suppositories	80 mg, 160 mg, 325 mg, 650 mg
	Tablets/caplets	325 mg, 500 mg, 625 mg
Ibuprofen	Capsule/tablet	100 mg (tablet only), 200 mg
	Chewable tablets	100 mg
	Liquids	50 mg/1.25 mL, 100 mg/5 mL, 200 mg/5 mL

Note: Doses bolded with asterisks (*) are recommended for that patient group, but given primarily with physician guidance.

Prepared by Mark Botti; updated by Kelly Shea and Jeanine Abrons

Pediatric Commercially Available Dosage Forms and Doses/Concentrations of Antihistamines

Cetirizine			Diphenhydramine		
Age	Dose (in milligrams [mg])	Dose (in milliliters [mL] of liquid)	Age (years)	Usual dose	Max daily dose
< 6 months	Not recommended	Not applicable	< 2	Not recommended	Not applicable
6 to 12 months	2.5 mg once daily	2.5 mg = 2.5 mL	2 to < 6	6.25 to 12.5 mg*	37.5 mg/day*
12 to 23 months	Initial: 2.5 mg once daily. May increase to 2.5 mg twice daily	2.5 mg = 2.5 mL	6 to 11	12.5 to 25 mg	150 mg/day
2 to 5 years	Initial: 2.5 mg once daily. May increase to 2.5 mg twice daily or 5 mg daily	5 mg = 5 mL	≥ 12	25 to 50 mg	300 mg/day
≥ 6 years	5 to 10 mg per day as one dose or divided into 2 doses	10 mg = 10 mL	*Doses for 2 to < 4 years should be given under physician guidance.* Dose is 5 mg/kg/day divided into 3 to 4 doses as needed or every 4 to 8 hours. Do not take more than 6 doses/day. Comes in alcohol-free, dye-free, sorbitol-free, & sugar-free options. Liquids available with cherry, fruit, berry, mango, & vanilla cherry. Strips are grape flavored. Tablets available as cherry & grape flavors.		
Solution and syrups available as a hydrochloride are available as a liquid preparation in grape, banana-grape, & bubble gum flavor. Solutions are often dye free, gluten free, & sugar free (verify with specific product). Chewable tablets are available as tutti-fruitti, grape, & citrus.					

Medication	Dosage Forms	Commercially Available Products
Cetirizine	Capsules/Dispersible Tablets	10 mg
	Chewable Tablets/Tablets	5 mg, 10 mg
	Liquid	5 mg/5 mL
Diphenhydramine	Capsules/Tablets	25 mg, 50 mg
	Chewable Tablets/Strips	12.5 mg
	Liquid	5 mg/5 mL, 12.5 mg/5 mL

Dosing Device	Advantages & Disadvantages	Comments
Medication cup	• Advantages: Ease of use • Disadvantages: Not accurate for small doses	• Cups from some products aren't the same
Dosing spoon/dropper	• Advantages: Ease of use • Disadvantage: Difficult to administer completely	• Check that liquid does not remain in spoon/dropper for accuracy
Dosing syringe	• Advantages: Accurate & complete dosing of liquids • Disadvantage: Patient familiarity	• Remove cap before use

Pediatric Commercially Available Dosage Forms and Doses/Concentrations of Antihistamines *(continued)*

Fexofenadine		Loratidine		
Age	**Dose (in milligrams [mg])**	**Age**	**Dose (in milligrams [mg])**	**Dose (in milliliters [mL] of liquid)**
≥ 6 months to < 2 years	< 10.5 kg: 15 mg BID > 10.5 kg: 30 mg BID	< 2 years	Not recommended	Not applicable
≥ 2 years to < 12 years	30 mg BID	2 to 5 years	5 mg once daily	5 mL
≥ 12 years	60 mg BID or 180 mg daily	≥ 6 years	10 mg once daily	10 mL
		Solution & syrups available as a hydrochloride are available as liquid preparations in grape, banana-grape, & fruit flavor. Chewable tablets available in grape flavor. Oral disintegrating tablets (ODT) available as bubblegum, citrus, & fruit flavors. Solutions are often alcohol free, dye free, gluten free, & sugar free (verify with specific product).		

Medication	Dosage Forms	Commercially Available Products
Fexofenadine	Tablet	60 mg, 180 mg
	Oral Disintegrating Tablet (ODT)	30 mg
	Suspension	30 mg/5 mL
Loratidine	Capsules/Tablets	10 mg
	Chewable Tablets	5 mg
	Dispersible Tablets	5 mg, 10 mg
	Liquids	5 mg/5 mL

Note: Doses bolded with asterisks (*) are recommended for that patient group, but given primarily with physician guidance.

Prepared by Mark Botti; updated by Kelly Shea

Pediatric Commercially Available Dosage Forms and Doses for Gastrointestinal or Motion Sickness Purposes

Simethicone for Gas & Bloating

Simethicone		
Age	**Dose (in milligrams [mg])**	**Dose (in milliliters [mL] of liquid)**
< 2 years	20	0.3
2 to 12 years	40	0.6
> 12 years	40 to 125; may give single dose of 500 mg; do not exceed 500 mg per day	Consider chewable tabs

Administer up to 4 times per day with meals.
Chewable tabs available in cherry crème, cool mint, peppermint, & peppermint crème. Strips available in cinnamon & peppermint. Suspension available in fruit & vanilla. Some formulations come alcohol free, dye free, &/or saccharin free.

Medication	Dosage Forms	Doses/Concentrations Available
Simethicone	Capsule	125 mg, 180 mg
	Chewable tablets	80 mg, 125 mg
	Liquids	20 mg/0.3 mL
	Strips	40 mg, 62.5 mg

Polyethylene Glycol (Miralax) for Constipation

Polyethylene Glycol: Miralax		
Age	**Dosing**	**Maximum Daily Dose**
6 months to 12 months	80 mg every 6 hours	320 mg/day
12 months to 3 years	80 mg every 4 to 6 hours	400 mg/day
> 3 years to 6 years	120 mg every 4 to 6 hours	600 mg/day
> 6 years to 12 years	325 mg every 4 to 6 hours	1625 mg/day
≥ 12 years	650 mg every 4 to 6 hours	3900 mg/day

Weight-based dosing is also available. Reference: Seattle Children's Hospital. Mild Constipation: Polyethylene glycol (Miralax) Dosage Table.

How to use Polyethylene Glycol Instructions for Mixing
- Use for 5 to 7 days. Note that it may take up to 7 days to see results.
- Mix with juice or water. Dissolve completely.
- Do not mix with milk, as the medicine does not work as well with dairy products.

Cautionary Notes
- Use the cap to measure the correct amount of medication.
- Stop the medicine if loose, watery, or liquid stools; if your child starts to vomit or develops bloody diarrhea or stomach pain.

Motion Sickness Medications

Motion Sickness Medications Pediatric Dosing		
Motion Sickness Medications	**Dosage Forms**	**Dosing**
Dimenhydrinate	Tablet: 50 mg Chewable: 50 mg	• 2 to 5 years: 12.5 to 25 mg every 6 to 8 hours (Maximum dosage = 150 mg/day) • 6 to 11 years: 25 to 50 mg every 6 to 8 hours (Maximum dosage = 150 mg/day) • ≥ 12 years: 50 to 100 mg every 4 to 6 hours (Maximum dosage = 400 mg/day)
Meclizine	Tablet: 12.5 mg, 25 mg, 50 mg Chewable: 25 mg	≥ 12 years: 25 to 50 mg 1 hour before travel, repeat every 24 hours as needed

Card by Jeanine P. Abrons and Mark Botti; updated by Jeanine P. Abrons & Kelly Shea

Use of Creams in Pediatric Populations

Hydrocortisone Cream		Diphenhydramine Cream		Bacitracin	
Age/Indication	**Dosing/Administration Notes**	**Age/Indication**	**Dosing/Administration Notes**	**Age/Indication**	**Dosing/Administration Notes**
Atopic dermatitis: Infants ≥ 3 months/ Children/ Adolescents	Apply a thin film to affected area twice daily; if no improvement in 2 weeks, reassess diagnosis	**Relief of pain/ itching:** Children ≥ 2 years/ Adolescents	Apply 1% or 2% concentration to affected area up to 3 to 4 times daily	**Prevention of infection:** Infants/Children/ Adolescents	Apply small amount 1 to 3 times daily; duration of therapy > 7 days is not recommended, unless directed by healthcare provider. Note: Do not use in the eyes or over large areas of the body.
Minor dermatologic irritation: Children ≥ 2 years/ Adolescents	Apply to affected area up to 3 to 4 times daily				
Avoid contact with eyes; Apply a thin film to clean, dry skin, and rub in gently. Do not apply to face, underarms, or groin unless directed by a physician. Do not occlude or wrap.		*Cream, gel: Apply thin coat to affected area; Stick: Holding stick straight down, press tip of stick on affected area repeatedly until liquid flows, then dab sparingly*		*Clean the affected area. Apply a small amount of product (an amount equal to the surface area of the tip of a finger); may cover with sterile bandage.*	

Note: Other indications for these creams exist; more common indications only were included; All are for external use only

Pediatric Measurements

Measuring Device	Size	Measure to Nearest
Oral syringe*	1 mL	0.02 mL
	3 mL	0.1 mL
	5 mL	0.2 mL
	10 mL	0.2 mL
Dosing spoon	10 mL	1 mL
Dosing cup	Variable	Check dosing cup

*Note: * = ISMP (Institute for Safe Medication Practices) only recommends use of oral syringes with metric doses. Other nonmetric syringes not recommended; N/A = not applicable.*

Prepared by Mark Botti

Inappropriate Medications in Older Adults

BEERS CRITERIA
The Beers Criteria for Potentially Inappropriate Medication Use in Older Adults was originally published in 1991. The most recent edition was released in 2019.[1] This update removes drugs no longer available, adds new drugs, & adds an expanded list of conditions considered. The new update also uses an evidence-based approach in developing the guidelines & a rating system for each criterion.

KEY POINTS
- The criteria are not meant to substitute for professional, clinical judgment, & therapy should be individualized for each patient.
- The criteria are meant to "inform clinical decision making, research, training, & policy to improve the quality/safety of prescribing medications for older adults."[1]
- The Screening Tool of Older Persons' Potentially Inappropriate Prescriptions & Screening Tool to Alert Doctors to the Right Treatment (STOPP/START criteria) should be used in a complementary manner to the Beers Criteria.[3]

ORGANIZATION/RESOURCE
The American Geriatrics Society (AGS) has a printable pocket card available for download on the organization's website for a fee.

Table #	2019 AGS Beers Criteria® Table Focus
Table 2	• Criteria by Organ System, Therapeutic Category & Drug(s)
Table 3	• Criteria Due to Drug-Disease or Drug Syndrome Interactions That May Exacerbate the Disease or Syndrome
Table 4	• Drugs to Be Used with Caution in Older Adults
Table 5	• Clinically Important Drug-Drug Interactions That Should Be Avoided in Older Adults
Table 6	• Medications That Should Be Avoided or Have Their Dosage Reduced with Varying Levels of Kidney Function in Older Adults
Table 7	• Drugs with Strong Anticholinergic Properties
Table 8	• Medications/Criteria Removed Since 2015
Table 9	• Medications/Criteria Added Since 2015
Table 10	• Medications/Criteria Modified Since 2015

OTHER INFORMATION
Most adverse drug events in older adults are attributed to a small number of medications. In a recent study, four medication classes were found to be responsible for most adverse effects in adults: warfarin, insulin, oral antiplatelet agents, & oral hypoglycemic agents.[2,3] Close monitoring of these medication classes should be employed to reduce patient risk. Criteria are not meant to apply at end of life or when a patient is receiving pain & palliative care where risk to benefit considerations may be different.[1]

REFERENCES
1. American Geriatrics Society 2019 Beers Criteria® Update Expert Panel. American Geriatrics Society Updated AGS Beers Criteria® for Potentially Inappropriate Medication Use in Older Adults. *J Am Geriatr Soc*, 2019 Apr. 67(4):674–94.
2. O'Mahony D, O'Sullivan D, Byrne S, et al. STOPP/START criteria for potentially inappropriate prescribing in older people: Version 2. *Age & Ageing*. 2015;44:213–18.
3. Budnitz DS, Lovegrove MC, Shehab N, Richards CL. Emergency Hospitalizations for adverse events in older Americans. *N Engl J Med*. 2011;365(21):2002.

Inappropriate Medications in Older Adults *(continued)*

Common Medications to Avoid in Older Adults	Additional Information
Aspirin	• Risk of major bleeding from aspirin increases in older age. • Cardiovascular risks may outweigh benefits. • Risk versus benefit in adults 70 years of age & older.
Nonsteroidal Anti-Inflammatory Drugs (NSAIDs)	• Avoid due to risk of indigestion, ulcers, & bleeding. • Shorter-acting versions are considered a safer choice. • May increase blood pressure, impair renal function, worsen heart failure. • Do not use in combination with other medications that increase risk of bleeding.
Certain Diabetes Drugs	• Certain antihyperglycemic medications, such as sulfonylureas may result in hypoglycemic episodes in older adults.
Certain Cardiovascular Drugs	• Digoxin: avoid doses > 0.125 mg, which can result in toxicity. • Certain blood pressure medications may increase risk of orthostatic hypotension or bradycardia. • Dabigatran & Rivaroxaban: ↑ caution over the age of 75. • Prasugrel: ↑ risk of bleeding in older adults; benefit in highest-risk older adults (e.g., those with prior myocardial infarction or diabetes mellitus) may offset risk • Other: warfarin, angiotensin-converting-enzyme inhibitors (ACEI); alpha-1 blockers; amiodarone; nifedipine; & others.
Muscle Relaxants	• Muscle relaxants can cause sedation, increased confusion, fall risk, constipation, dry mouth, & urinary retention. • Examples include cyclobenzaprine & methocarbamol.
Medications for Anxiety/Insomnia/Depression	• Medications for anxiety and insomnia can ↑ risk of falls & confusion. • Mirtazapine, Serotonin-Norepinephrine Reuptake Inhibitor (SNRIs), Selective Serotonin Reuptake Inhibitor (SSRIs) & Tricyclic Antidepressants (TCAs): may exacerbate or cause SIADH or hyponatremia; monitor sodium level closely
Certain Anticholinergic Drugs	• Anticholinergic drugs may result in confusion, constipation, urinary retention, blurred vision, & hypotension. • Examples may include certain antidepressants, certain anti-Parkinson drugs, trihexyphenidyl, dicyclomine, & oxybutynin.
Meperidine	• This medication may increase risk of confusion & seizures.
Certain Antihistamine Medications	• Certain antihistamines may result in confusion, constipation, urinary retention, blurred vision, & dry mouth.
Antipsychotics (for indications other than psychosis)	• Haloperidol, risperidone, & quetiapine are antipsychotic medications that may result in increased risk of stroke, movement disorders (such as tremors), and falls. • May exacerbate or cause SIADH or hyponatremia; monitor sodium level closely when starting or changing dosages in older adults
Estrogens	• Estrogens ↑ older adults' risk for clots & lack cognitive preventative effects. • May increase risk for breast and endometrial cancers.

References: Information adapted from Ten Medications Older Adults Should Avoid or Use with Caution. Healthinaging.org: Trusted Information. Better Care by the American Geriatrics Foundation for Health in Aging. Full content available at: https://www.healthinaging.org/tools-and-tips/ten-medications-older-adults-should-avoid-or-use-caution (Accessed November 2021; Table 4. 2019 American Geriatrics Society Beers Criteria® for Potentially Inappropriate Medications: Drugs To Be Used With Caution in Older Adults).

Brief Overview of STOPP/START Criteria
- **STOPP** (screening tool of older people's prescriptions): 80 clinically significant criteria for potentially inappropriate medication use (drug and disease interactions, therapeutic duplication)
- **START** (screening tool to alert to right treatment): 34 common disease states in older adults where medications are indicated (evidence based)
- Organized as analgesic, cardiovascular, central nervous system, endocrine, gastrointestinal, respiratory, & urinary tract drugs.

Prepared by Jeanine P. Abrons; updated by Erika Bethhauser, Thomas Roberts, Ashley Behrens, and Jeanine Abrons

Pregnancy and Lactation Resources: Medication-Related Resources

Name of Resource	How to Access	Description
Briggs' Drugs in Pregnancy & Lactation, Eleventh Edition	Wolters Kluwer Health/Lippincott Williams and Wilkins Textbook; Partial (preview) version available as free download at iTunes Store	• Summarizes known/possible side effects of medications in pregnancy and possibility of passage through breast milk when nursing; A to Z searchable index • Includes generic name; pharmacological class; risk factor; fetal risk summary; breast feeding summary; references
Centers for Disease Control (CDC) Treating for Two: Safer Medication Use In Pregnancy	https://www.cdc.gov/pregnancy/meds/treatingfortwo/index.html (Accessed 2021)	• This website provides general discussion points to use with patients for safer use of medicines during pregnancy. • Additional tabs include some guidelines/recommendations by condition; multimedia/tools; key findings; & research.
Hale's Medication & a Mother's Milk	Overview: https://www.halesmeds.com/ (Accessed 2021)	• Includes recommendations by the American Academy of Pediatrics • Also includes, for 1,300 herbals, prescription, over-the-counter (OTC), & street drugs—drug name/generic name; uses; drug monograph (understood knowledge of the drug; ability to enter breastmilk; time-dependent concentration; other clinically relevant information); pregnancy & lactation risk category; theoretical/relative infant dose; adult/pediatric concerns; drug interactions; alternatives; pharmacokinetic/pharmacodynamics information
Infant Risk Center	http://www.infantrisk.com (Accessed 2021)	• Provided by Texas Tech University Health Sciences Center • Tabs on Pregnancy & Breastfeeding • Apps available: MommyMeds for Mothers & InfantRisk Center for Health Providers
LactMed (Drugs & Lactation Database)	http://toxnet.nlm.nih.gov/newtoxnet/lactmed.htm (Accessed 2021)	• "The LactMed® database contains information on drugs & other chemicals to which breastfeeding mothers may be exposed." • <u>Components listed:</u> Levels anticipated; effects in breastfed infants; effects on lactation & breast milk; alternatives to consider; references • Updated monthly
Mother to Baby	http://www.mothertobaby.org	Facts sheets for patients & healthcare providers by specialty, condition, & medication.
Reprotox	https://reprotox.org/	Gives summaries of the effects of medications, chemicals, infections, and physical agents on pregnancy, reproduction, & development.
Consult multiple resources, as recommendations may differ.		

Known Teratogens
Alcohol; angiotensin-converting-enzyme inhibitors (ACEI); angiotensin receptor blockers (ARBs); carbamazepine; cocaine; coumarin anticoagulants; diethylstilbestrol (DES); methotrexate; phenytoin; isotretinoin; lithium; misoprostol; statins; tetracyclines; thalidomide; valproate

Griffin BL, Stone RH, El-Ibiary SY, Westberg S, Shealy K, Forinash A, Yancey A, Vest K, Karaoui LR, Rafie S, Horlen C. Guide for drug selection during pregnancy and lactation: What pharmacists need to know for current practice. *Annals of Pharmacotherapy*. 2018 Aug;52(8):810–8; Ledan SH. OTC Medication Use in Pregnancy & Breastfeeding. US Pharmacist, September 17, 2019: https://www.uspharmacist.com/article/otc-medication-use-in-pregnancy-and-breastfeeding (Accessed November 2021)

Prepared by Jeanine P. Abrons

Pregnancy Risk Classifications

Pregnancy & Lactation Labeling Final Rule (PLLR)	
For prescription drugs submitted after 2015, the following information is provided in replacement of the pregnancy letter categories (the previous system was to be removed by June 2018).	
Pregnancy (includes labor & delivery)	<ul><li>Provides information about dosing/risk to developing fetus as well as registry information to monitor data on impacts to pregnant women</li><li>Subsections are excluded if no data is available with the exception of the Risk Summary section.</li><li>Pregnancy Exposure Registry Information</li><li>Risk Summary</li><li>Clinical Considerations</li><li>Available Data</li></ul>
Lactation (includes nursing mothers)	<ul><li>Includes drugs that should not be used during breastfeeding, known human/animal data, clinical effects on infant, pharmacokinetics, risk/benefits & timing to minimize exposure</li><li>Risk Summary</li><li>Clinical Considerations</li><li>Data</li></ul>
Females & Males of Reproductive Potential	<ul><li>Includes testing information or birth control before, during & after medications as well as medication effects on fertility/pregnancy loss</li><li>Pregnancy Testing</li><li>Contraception</li></ul>

Reference: https://www.drugs.com/pregnancy-categories.html#:~:text=In%201979%2C%20the%20FDA%20established, defects%20if%20used%20during%20pregnancy (Accessed 2021)

Prepared by Jeanine P. Abrons

Safe and Unsafe Use of OTC Medications during Pregnancy - Various Conditions

- Non-pharmacologic therapies should be prioritized over pharmacologic therapies.
- Each individual pregnant person may have a different threshold for safety.
- Pregnant individuals should be encouraged to discuss any medication use with their OB/midwife.

Common Conditions	UNSAFE OTC Treatments During Pregnancy: Trimester UNSAFE to Use	SAFE OTC Treatments During Pregnancy: Trimester SAFE to Use
Allergic Rhinitis	See Safe to Use Column (encourage discussion with OB or midwife)	• Chlorpheniramine: all trimesters • Diphenhydramine (Benadryl®): all trimesters • Cromolyn (NasalCrom®): all trimesters • Saline nasal spray/irrigation: all trimesters • Fluticasone nasal spray (Flonase®): all trimesters • 2nd generation antihistamines – Cetirizine (Zyrtec®), Loratadine (Claritin®), Fexofenadine (Allegra®)**: all trimesters
Congestion	• Phenylephrine: avoid as OTC, particularly 1st trimester • Pseudoephedrine: 1st trimester	• Nasal saline sprays: all trimesters • Adhesive nasal strips: all trimesters • Use of humidifier: all trimesters
Cough	• Codeine: all trimesters (especially 1st, 3rd)	• Guaifenesin: all trimesters • Dextromethorphan*: all trimesters
Pain, Fever, and Headache	• Aspirin: avoid high dose in 1st & 3rd trimesters[a] • Aspirin/acetaminophen/caffeine (Excedrin): do not use • Ibuprofen/Naproxen: avoid in 1st & 3rd trimesters	• Acetaminophen*: DOC: all trimesters
Fungal Infections/ Dermatitis	See Safe to Use Column (encourage discussion with OB or midwife)	• Nasal hydrocortisone*: all trimesters • Topical antifungals (prefer over oral): clotrimazole/miconazole: all trimesters
Dermatologic Disorders/Acne	• Retinoids/retinol: do not use	• Benzoyl peroxide; DOC: all trimesters • Salicylic acid*: all trimesters • Glycolic acid: all trimesters

APhA

Safe and Unsafe Use of OTC Medications during Pregnancy - Gastrointestinal Medications

Common Conditions	UNSAFE OTC Treatments During Pregnancy: Trimester UNSAFE to Use	SAFE OTC Treatments During Pregnancy: Trimester SAFE to Use
Nausea	See Safe to Use Column (encourage discussion with OB or midwife)	• Ginger^: all trimesters • Pyroxidine (Vitamin B6)^: all trimesters • Doxylamine: all trimesters • Additional antihistamines (meclizine, dimenhydrinate, diphenhydramine)**: all trimesters
Heartburn	See Safe to Use Column (encourage discussion with OB or midwife)	• Calcium carbonate; DOC: all trimesters • Antacids* with Al–, Ca2+, Mg2+: all trimesters
Diarrhea	• Bismuth subsalicylate (Pepto-Bismol®): do not use, particularly in the 1st and 3rd trimesters • Loperamide** (Imodium®): 1st	• Oral rehydration solution (ORS)
Constipation	• Castor oil: do not use • Mineral oil: do not use	• Polyethylene glycol 3350 (Miralax®); DOC: all trimesters • Colace/Sodium Docusate: all trimesters • Fiber supplements (Metamucil®, Citrucel®, Fibercon®, Benefiber®): all trimesters • Sennosides/bisocodyl**: all trimesters

Notes: DOC = drug of choice

* recommend lowest strength for shortest time possible; ** = likely safe but other equivalent choices have more data; ^ = herbal/vitamin supplement.

* be used to reduce the risk of pre-eclampsia at low doses under the guidance of a physician or midwife

This table is for general information. Always have patients discuss medications & supplements with a physician or midwife. Generally, medications under "UNSAFE" have specifically been stated in literature to use with caution, to avoid in certain trimesters, to have limited human data, or to have better alternatives. Medications under "SAFE" are either DOCs, have not been cautioned for use, or do not have specific restrictions documented in literature.

References: (Accessed January 2022)

Body, C., and J.A. Christie. "Gastrointestinal diseases in pregnancy." Gastroenterology Clinical of North America 45, no. 2(2016): 267–83.

Briggs, G., R. Freeman, C. Towers, and A. Forninash. Drugs in Pregnancy and Lactation: A Reference Guide to Fetal and Neonatal Risk. Philadelphia, PA: Wolters Kluwer Health, 2017.

Chien, A.L., J. Qi, B. Rainer, et al. "Treatment of acne in pregnancy." Journal of the American Board of Family Medicine 29 (2016): 254–62.

Kuston, C.A., and D.M. Elston. "Treatment of common skin infections and infestations during pregnancy." Dermatologic Therapy 26 (2013): 312–20.

Larson, L.E., and T.M. File. "Treatment of respiratory infections in pregnant patients." UpToDate. Accessed January 3, 2022. https://www.uptodate.com/contents/treatment-of-respiratory-infections-in-pregnant-patients.

Schatz, M. "Recognition and management of allergic disease during pregnancy." UpToDate. Accessed January 3, 2022. https://www.uptodate.com/contents/recognition-and-management-of-allergic-disease-during-pregnancy.

Smith, J.A., K.A. Fox, and S.M. Clark. "Nausea and vomiting of pregnancy: Treatment and outcome." UpToDate. Accessed January 24, 2022. https://www.uptodate.com/contents/nausea-and-vomiting-of-pregnancy-treatment-and-outcome.

Prepared by Brittany Hayes; updated by Jeanine P. Abrons, Lauren Jonkman, Andrew La, and Randall Bendis

Immunization Schedule for Children and Adolescent Ages 18 Years or Younger

Vaccine	Dose/Recommended Ages for All Children	Recommended Catch-up Immunization	Other/Notes
Hepatitis B (HepB)	• 1st dose: Birth • 2nd dose: 1 month to 2 months • 3rd dose: 6 to 8 months	• Unvaccinated persons should complete a 3-dose series at 0, 1 to 2, & 6 months • Adolescents age 11 to 15 years may use an alternative 2-dose schedule with at least 4 months between doses (adult form Recombivax HB only) • Adolescents age 18 years or older may receive a 2-dose series of HepB (Heplisav-B) at least 4 weeks apart • Adolescents age 18 years or older may receive the combined Hep A & Hep B vaccine (Twinrix) at 0, 1 & 6 months or 4-dose series at 0, 7 & 21 to 30 days then a booster at 12 months	• Minimum age: birth (monovalent HepB vaccine only); timing of dosing depends on weight of infant & whether mom is HBsAg(−), (+), or status is unknown; see footnotes for guidance** • Minimum interval between doses 1 & 2 = 4 weeks • Minimum interval between doses 2 & 3 = 8 weeks (16 weeks after 1st dose; when 4 doses are administered) • Minimum age for third or fourth = 24 weeks • Revaccination not for persons with normal immune status vaccinated as infants, children, adolescents, or adults • Consider revaccination for infants born to HBsAg-positive mothers, hemodialysis patients & other immunocompromised patients
Rotavirus (RV)	• Rotarix: 2-dose series at 2 & 4 months • RotaTeq: 3-dose series at 2, 4 & 6 months • If any dose is RotaTeq or unknown: default to 3-dose series	• Do not start the series on or after age 15 weeks, 0 days. • 8 months = max age for final dose • Dose 1 to 2 & 2 to 3: 4 week interval	• Minimum age 6 weeks for both vaccines
Diphtheria, tetanus, & acellular pertussis (DTaP)	• 1st dose: 2 months • 2nd dose: 4 months • 3rd dose: 6 months • 4th dose: 15 to 18 months • 5th dose: 4 to 6 years	• 9 months to 4 years • 5th dose not needed if 4th dose given at ≥ age 4	• Minimum age: 6 weeks (4 years for Kinrix or Quadracel) • Prospectively: Administer dose 4 as early as 12 months if at least 6 months has passed since dose 3 • Retrospectively: If dose 4 was inadvertently administered early at 12 months it may be counted if at least 4 months since dose 3 • Wound management in < 7 years old with history of 3+ doses of tetanus-toxoid-containing vaccine: For all wounds (except clean/minor ones), give DTaP if > 5 years since last dose

Note: Coronavirus-19 Vaccine: See CDC for currently dosing/schedules as this is frequently changing. * = 3 dose and 4 dose series available; timing of a booster dose depends on whether child received primary series in the first year of life; http://www.immunize.org/askexperts/experts_hib.asp; https://www.cdc.gov/vaccines/hcp/vis/vis-statements/hib.html; ** = https://www.cdc.gov/vaccines/schedules/downloads/child/0-18yrs-child-combined-schedule.pdf (Accessed January 2021)

Prepared by Jeanine P. Abrons and Elisha Andreas

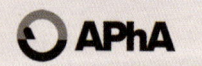

Immunization Schedule for Children and Adolescent Ages 18 Years or Younger *(continued)*

Vaccine	Dose/Recommended Ages for All Children	Recommended Catch-up Immunization	Other/Notes
Haemophilus influenza type b (Hib) ActHIB, Hiberix, Pentacel: 4-dose series; PedvaxHIB: 3-dose series	• 1st dose: 2 months • 2nd dose: 4 months • 3rd dose: 6 months (if using 4-dose series only) • 4th dose: Age 12 to 15 months	Based on first dose: • @ age 7 to 11 mo: Give 2nd dose greater than or equal to 4 weeks later; 3rd dose at 12 to 15 mo or 8 weeks after dose 2 (whichever is longer) • @ age 12 to 14 mo: Give 2nd dose greater than or equal to 8 weeks after dose 1 • @ > 12 mo & before 15 mo: Give 3rd dose 8 weeks after dose 2 • 2 doses of PedvaxHIB before 12 mo: Give 3rd dose at 12 to 59 mo & 8 weeks after dose 2 • 1 dose at 15 mo or > or not vaccinated age 60 months or older who are not high risk: No more doses • Unvaccinated at 15 to 59 mo: Give 1 dose	• Minimum age = 6 weeks • Special situations with additional dosing include chemotherapy or radiation treatment, hematopoietic stem cell transplant (HSCT), anatomic or functional asplenia (including sickle cell disease), elective splenectomy, HIV infection, immunoglobulin deficiency & early component complement deficiency • For minimum intervals between doses, refer to cdc.gov

Pneumococcal conjugate (PCV13) or PPSV23	• 1st dose: 2 months
	• 2nd dose: 4 months
	• 3rd dose: 6 months
	• 4th dose: 12 to 15 months
		• PCV13 Catch-up: 1 dose for healthy kids age 24 to 59 months with incomplete PCV13 series; see CDC for other catch-up guidance (Table 2)	• Minimum age for PCV13 = 6 weeks; minimum age for PPSV23 = 2 years
			• For certain high-risk groups: refer to cdc.gov
			• Special situations for dosing:
			  ○ When both PCV13 & PPSV23 are indicated: give PCV13 first; do not give both at same visit
			  ○ Chronic heart disease, chronic lung disease (including asthma treated with high-dose oral corticosteroids) & diabetes
			  ○ Cerebrospinal fluid leak, cochlear implant
			  ○ Sickle cell disease/hemoglobinopathies; immunodeficiency; HIV; chronic renal failure; nephrotic syndrome; malignant neoplasms/leukemias; lymphomas; Hodgkin disease; immunosuppressive drug/radiation therapy; solid organ transplantation; multiple myeloma
			  ○ Chronic liver disease, alcoholism

Note: Coronavirus-19 Vaccine: See CDC for currently dosing/schedules as this is frequently changing. * = 3 dose and 4 dose series available; timing of a booster dose depends on whether child received primary series in the first year of life: http://www.immunize.org/askexperts/experts_hib.asp; https://www.cdc.gov/vaccines/hcp/vis/vis-statements/hib.html; ** = https://www.cdc.gov/vaccines/schedules/downloads/child/0-18yrs-child-combined-schedule.pdf (Accessed January 2021)

Prepared by Jeanine P. Abrons and Elisha Andreas

Immunization Schedule for Children and Adolescent Ages 18 Years or Younger *(continued)*

Vaccine	Dose/Recommended Ages for All Children	Recommended Catch-up Immunization	Other/Notes
Inactivated poliovirus (IPV < 18 years)	• 1st dose: 2 months • 2nd dose: 4 months • 3rd dose: 6 months to 18 months • 4th dose: 4 to 6 years	• In the first 6 months of life: See minimum ages only if travel to polio-edemic region or with an outbreak • Note that an Oral Polio Vaccine (OPV) is available with different dosing & with mixed OPV-IPV dosing	• Minimum age = 6 weeks; Maximum age = 18 • Administer final dose at or after age 4 years & at least 6 months after previous dose • 4 or more doses of IPV can be administered before age 4 when a combo vaccination is used. Dose still recommended on or after 4 years & at least 6 months after prior dose
Influenza (IIV)	• Annual: Administer starting at 6 months	• N/A	• For children age 6 months thru 8 years who received < 2 doses before July 1, 2020, or children whose vaccination history is unknown: Administer 2 doses separated by at least 4 weeks • Children 6 to 8 years and older than 8 years: only 1 dose is required (who received at 2 or > doses before July 1, 2020) • Special situations with dosing on CDC website: egg allergy (with hives only or with other symptoms), situations where LAIV4 is not recommended
Measles, mumps, rubella (MMR)	• 2 dose series: 12 months thru 15 months • 2nd dose: 4 to 6 years (may be given as early as 4 weeks after dose 1)	• Unvaccinated children & adolescents: 2-dose series at least 4 weeks apart	• Minimum age = 12 months; Maximum age for MMRV = 12 years • Ensure that all school aged children & adolescents get • See travel card for travel related guidance separate dosing for infants age 6 to 11 mo & unvaccinated children greater than or equal to age 12 mo
Varicella (VAR)	• 1st dose: 12 thru 15 months • 2nd dose: 4 to 6 years	• Age 7 to 12 years: Routine interval: 3 months (dose administered after 4-week interval may be counted) • Age 13 & older: Routine interval: 4 to 8 weeks (minimum interval = 4 weeks)	• Minimum age = 12 months; Maximum age for MMRV = 12 years • 2nd dose may be given as early as 3 months after dose 1 (dose administered after a 4-week interval may be counted) • Minimum interval between dose 1 & 2 if < 13 years: 3 months • Minimum interval between dose 1 & 2 if >13 years: 4 weeks
Hepatitis A (HepA)	• 2-dose series: Beginning at age 12 months to 23 months	• Unvaccinated persons through age 18: complete 2-dose series • Persons who previously received 1 dose at age 12 months or older should receive dose 2 at least 6 months later • Adolescents 18 years & older: May get combined HepA/HepB vaccine (Twinrix) as 3-dose series (0, 1 & 6 months) or 4 dose series (0, 7, 21 to 30 days, followed by a dose at 12 monts**h**)	• Minimum age: 12 months • Minimum interval between doses = 6 months • See travel medicine card for persons traveling to countries with high or intermediate endemic Hepatitis A separate doses available for infants 6 to 11 mo & unvaccinated age greater than or equal to 12 mo

Note: ** = https://www.cdc.gov/vaccines/schedules/hcp/imz/child-adolescent.html#note-hepa (Accessed 2021)

Immunization Schedule for Children and Adolescent Ages 18 Years or Younger *(continued)*

Vaccine	Dose/Recommended Ages for All Children	Information Related to Catch-up Immunization/Other Notes
Serogroup A,C,W,Y meningococcal vaccine*	1st dose: 11 to 12 years 2nd dose: 16 years	• Minimum age: 2 months (MenACWY-CRM Menveo), 9 months (MenACWY-D Menactra); 2 years (MenACWY-TT, MenQuadfi) • Age 13 to 15 years: 1 dose now & booster at age 16 to 18 years. Minimum interval 8 weeks • Age 16 to 18 years: 1 dose • Menactra should be given either before or at the same time as DTaP & must be administered at least 4 weeks after end of PCV13 series • Special dosing for anatomic or functional asplenia, HIV infection, persistent complement component deficiency, eculizumab use, travel in countries with hyperendemic or epidemic meningococcal disease and 1st year college students who live in residential housing or military recruits: refer to CDC website • Minimum interval between dose 1 & 2 = 8 weeks • Different from serogroup B vaccine
Tetanus, diphtheria, & acellular pertussis (DTaP)	5-dose series: 1st dose: 2 months 2nd dose: 4 months 3rd dose: 6 months 4th dose: 15 to 18 months 5th dose: 4 to 6 years	• Prospective routine vaccination: dose 4 can be given as early as 12 months > 6 months after dose 3 • Retrospective routine vaccination: 4th dose inadvertently given at 12 months may be counted if 4 months since 3rd dose • Catch-up dose 5 not necessary if 4th dose given at age 4 or older & 6 months after dose 3 • Special situations include wound management in children less than age 7 with 3 or more prior doses of tetanus-toxoid-containing vaccine
Human papillomavirus	• Routine vaccination for ages 11 to 12, may start at age 9; Give series on schedule of 0, 6 to 12 months; can start at age 9 interval = 5 months, repeat if dose too soon • Administer thru age 18 • 1st dose before age 15: 2 doses on schedule of 0, 6 to 12 months; minimum interval = 5 months • 1st dose at or after age 15: 3 doses on schedule of 0, 1 to 2, 6 months	• Vaccine dose administered at shorter intervals than minimum 2-dose schedule interval • Minimum age of 9 for routine/catch-up doses • Number of recommended doses based on age of administration of 1st dose • If vaccine administered on shorter interval than recommended, re-administer after minimum interval has been met • Age 15 years or older at initiation: 3-dose series minimum intervals: 4 weeks between 1st & 2nd dose; 12 weeks between 2nd & 3rd dose; 5 months between 1st & 3rd dose • See CDC site for special populations**

Note: *For meningococcal B vaccination pneumococcal polysaccharide (PPSV23), see CDC website for use in high-risk conditions & other persons at increased risk of disease.   ** = https://www.cdc.gov/vaccines/schedules/hcp/child-adolescent.html (Accessed 2022).

Prepared by Jeanine P. Abrons and Elisha Andreas

Immunizations by Age for First Year of Life

Age	Immunizations to Be Given During Normal Dosing Schedule	Immunizations to Be Given During Normal Dosing Schedule	Needle Length/Injection Site
Birth	Hepatitis B*		Intramuscular: 5/8"; anterolateral thigh muscle; use 22- to 25-gauge needle
1 month	Hepatitis B (or month 2)*		
2 months	• Diphtheria, tetanus, & acellular pertussis (DTaP < 7 years)* • Hepatitis B (or month 1) (2nd dose if not given at month 1)* • Haemophilus influenza type b (1st dose)* • Inactivated poliovirus (IPV < 18 years) (1st dose)	• Pneumococcal conjugate (PCV13) (1st dose)* • Rotavirus (1st dose)**	Subcutaneous: 5/8" fatty tissue over anterolateral thigh muscle; use 23- to 25-gauge needle Intramuscular: 1" in anterolateral thigh muscle; use 22- to 25-gauge needle
4 months	• Rotavirus (2nd dose)** • Diphtheria, tetanus, & acellular pertussis (DTaP < 7 years)* • Haemophilus influenza type b (2nd dose)* • Pneumococcal conjugate (PCV13) (2nd dose)*	• Inactivated poliovirus (IPV < 18 years) (2nd dose)* • Catch-up immunization potential: Hepatitis B*	
6 months	• Diphtheria, tetanus, & acellular pertussis (DTaP < 7 years)* • Haemophilus influenza type b (if 3 or 4 dose series)* • Hepatitis B (potentially) 3rd dose may be given 6 months on* • Inactivated poliovirus (IPV < 18 years) 3rd dose may be given 6 months on*	• Influenza (annually; potential)** • Pneumococcal conjugate (PCV13) (3rd dose)* • Rotavirus (if 3-dose series)**	
9 months	• Hepatitis B (potentially) If 3rd dose not already given* • Inactivated poliovirus (IPV < 18 years) (potentially) If 3rd dose not already given* • Influenza (annually; potential)**	• Catch-up immunization potential: diphtheria, tetanus, & acellular pertussis (DTaP < 7 years)*, haemophilus* influenza type b; pneumococcal conjugate (PCV13)* • Certain high-risk groups: measles, mumps, rubella (MMR)***	
12 months	• Hepatitis B (potentially) If 3rd dose not already given* • Haemophilus influenza type b (if 3 or 4 dose series)* • Inactivated poliovirus (IPV < 18 years) if 3rd dose not already given* • Influenza (annually; potential)** • Measles, mumps, rubella (MMR)***	• Hepatitis A (potentially)* • Pneumococcal conjugate (PCV13) (potentially 4th dose)* • Varicella (potentially 1st dose)*** • Catch-up immunization potential: diphtheria, tetanus, & acellular pertussis (DTaP < 7 years)*	

Notes: * = dose or route of administration & dose dependent upon product; *** = Dose intramuscularly (IM) or subcutaneously (IM or subcutaneously of 0.5 mL; + = Dose subcutaneously of 0.5 mL. References: with https://www.cdc.gov/vaccines/schedules/downloads/child/0-18yrs-child-combined-schedule.pdf; immunize.org (Accessed 2022)

Prepared by Jeanine P. Abrons and Elisha Andreas

2021 Recommended Immunizations for Children from Birth Through 6 Years Old

Birth	1 month	2 months	4 months	6 months	12 months	15 months	18 months	19–23 months	2–3 years	4–6 years
HepB	HepB				HepB					
		RV	RV	RV						
		DTaP	DTaP	DTaP		DTaP				DTaP
		Hib	Hib	Hib	Hib					
		PCV13	PCV13	PCV13	PCV13					
		IPV	IPV	IPV		IPV				IPV
					MMR					MMR
					Varicella					Varicella
					HepA§					
				Influenza (Yearly)*						

Shaded boxes indicate the vaccine can be given during shown age range.

Is your family growing? To protect your new baby and yourself against whooping cough, get a Tdap vaccine. The recommended time is the 27th through 36th week of pregnancy. Talk to your doctor for more details.

NOTE:
If your child misses a shot, you don't need to start over, just go back to your child's doctor for the next shot. Talk with your child's doctor if you have questions about vaccines.

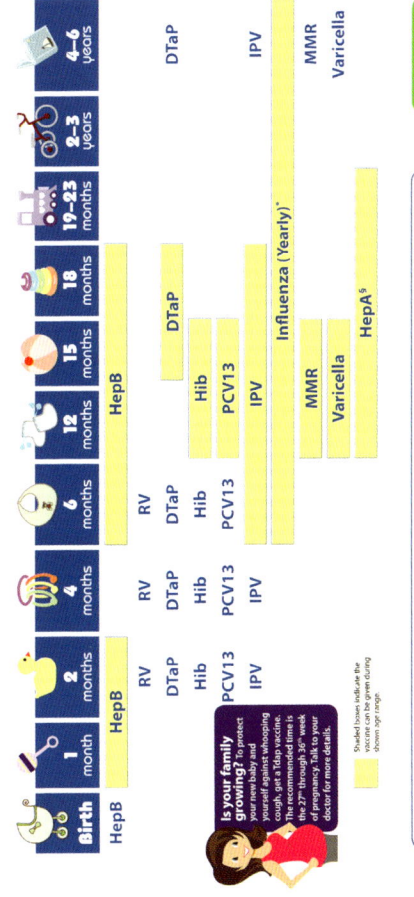

FOOTNOTES:
* Two doses given at least four weeks apart are recommended for children aged 6 months through 8 years of age who are getting an influenza (flu) vaccine for the first time and for some other children in this age group.
§ Two doses of HepA vaccine are needed for lasting protection. The first dose of HepA vaccine should be given between 12 months and 23 months of age. The second dose should be given 6 months after the last dose. HepA vaccination may be given to any child 12 months and older to protect against HepA. Children and adolescents who did not receive the HepA vaccine and are at high-risk, should be vaccinated against HepA.

If your child has any medical conditions that put him at risk for infection or is traveling outside the United States, talk to your child's doctor about additional vaccines that he may need.

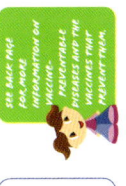

For more information, call toll free 1-800-CDC-INFO (1-800-232-4636) or visit www.cdc.gov/vaccines/parents

U.S. Department of Health and Human Services
Centers for Disease Control and Prevention

AMERICAN ACADEMY OF FAMILY PHYSICIANS
STRONG MEDICINE FOR AMERICA

SEE BACK PAGE FOR MORE INFORMATION ON VACCINE-PREVENTABLE DISEASES AND THE VACCINES THAT PREVENT THEM.

American Academy of Pediatrics
DEDICATED TO THE HEALTH OF ALL CHILDREN

Content source: National Center for Immunization and Respiratory Diseases.
Reference: https://www.cdc.gov/vaccines/parents/downloads/parent-ver-sch-0-6yrs.pdf (Accessed January 2022)

Travel Immunization and Travel Health Card—
ROUTINE VACCINATIONS

ROUTINE VACCINATIONS

Routine vaccines warrant special attention when a patient plans to travel. Ensure that all patients are up to date on routine adult or age-appropriate pediatric vaccines (e.g., influenza (yearly), varicella, MMR, polio, and others). To access the age-appropriate schedule for routine vaccines, please visit the Centers for Disease Control and Prevention (CDC) website: https://wwwnc.cdc.gov/travel/page/routine-vaccines. Routine vaccines with travel-specific indications or considerations are discussed next. Use of CDC catch-up immunization schedule may be necessary for pediatric patients who are un/under-vaccinated.

	VACCINE	INDICATION OR WHEN TO CONSIDER USING & DESCRIPTION
1	**HEPATITIS A VACCINE**	For all susceptible persons traveling to or working in countries that have high or intermediate rates of hepatitis A before traveling. • Children 6 to 11 months should be protected when traveling outside the USA to an area of risk. This dose should be in addition to the routine recommended two-dose schedule. • Unvaccinated children ages ≥ 1 year can receive the age-appropriate dose of hepatitis A vaccine as soon as travel is considered. • The initial dose of vaccine along with IM immune globulin at a separate injection site is recommended for the following travelers who are planning to depart to an area of risk in < 2 weeks: adults aged ≥ 40 years, immunocompromised people, people with chronic liver disease, and people with other chronic medical conditions. • Persons who are unable to receive the hepatitis A vaccine, including those who are allergic to the vaccine and children < 6 months, should receive a single dose of immune globulin, which provides up to two months of protection.
2	**HEPATITIS B VACCINE**	For all unvaccinated people traveling to areas with intermediate to high prevalence of chronic hepatitis B (HBsAg prevalence ≥ to 2%). • Vaccination to prevent hepatitis B may be considered for all international travelers, regardless of destination, depending on the traveler's behavioral risk or chronic disease diagnosis. • Recombinant hepatitis B vaccination should begin ≥6 months before travel so full three-dose vaccine series can be completed before departure. ○ An accelerated dosing schedule may be considered for patients at significant risk if there is not sufficient time to complete the series prior to departure. ○ For lower-risk patients, one or two doses may be administered prior to departure, but optimal protection is reliable only after complete series. ○ Adult patients receiving hemodialysis or with other immunocompromising conditions: consult package insert for dosing. • Adjuvanted hepatitis B vaccine is only for adults ≥18 years of age. ○ Two-dose series if ≥ 4 weeks apart (*both doses must be adjuvant formulation, if not, a three-dose series may be necessary*). ○ There may be diminished immune response in immunocompromised patients.
3	**MENINGOCOCCAL VACCINE**	For all patients who travel to countries where the disease is endemic or epidemic, including the sub-Saharan Africa meningitis belt during dry season (December to June). Proof of vaccination within three years for polysaccharide or within five years for the conjugated vaccine is required for entry into Saudi Arabia when traveling to Mecca during Hajj and Umrah pilgrimages. • Administer a single dose of MenACWY vaccine; then revaccinate with MenACWY vaccine every five years if increased risk of infection remains. • Infants and children who received Hib-MenCY-TT are not protected against serogroups A & W and should receive the quadrivalent vaccine before travel to highly endemic areas. • Children who received the last dose at < 7 years of age should receive an additional dose of MenACWY three years after their last dose. MenB vaccine is not recommended as a travel vaccine due to the low risk of meningococcal disease caused by serogroup B in these countries, unless the patient is believed to be at high risk for another reason (e.g., international exchange students in dorms/hostels or military barracks), in which case ACIP recommends shared clinical decision making to determine if the vaccine is warranted.

Created & updated by the APhA-APPM Immunizing Pharmacists Special Interest Group (SIG)

Travel Immunization and Travel Health Card—
ROUTINE VACCINATIONS *(continued)*

	VACCINE	INDICATION OR WHEN TO CONSIDER USING & DESCRIPTION

4	SARS-CoV-2 VACCINE	For age-appropriate approved patients in the USA traveling domestically or internationally. Please check updates as recommendations are changing frequently.
		• Coronavirus disease (COVID-19) is an infectious disease caused by the SARS-CoV-2 virus. It can spread from person to person, and the severity of the disease varies by individual and their underlying health conditions.
		• mRNA vaccines:
		  ○ Comirnaty (Pfizer BioNTech mRNA COVID-19 vaccine, BNT162b2)
		    ▪ As of November 2021, this is approved for ages ≥ 12 with emergency use authorization in ages 5 to 11.
		    ▪ ≥12 years of age: two-dose series 0.3 mL IM administered 21 days apart.
		    ▪ 5 to 11 years of age: two-dose series of 0.2 mL IM administered 21 days apart. (The adult product should not be used for children ages 5 to 11 years of age—it has unique packaging/dose).
		  ○ Guidelines are as of November 2021 and are changing rapidly. ***Please see the CDC website for current guidelines.***
		  ○ Moderna mRNA COVID-19 Vaccine (mRNA-1273)
		    ▪ Two-dose series of 0.5 mL IM administered 28 days apart.
		    ▪ FDA emergency use authorization for adults ≥ 18 years of age.
		  ○ Boosters of mRNA COVID-19 Vaccine are recommended for everyone ≥18 years as a single dose at least five months after completing the primary dose.
		    ▪ Any of the COVID-19 vaccines authorized are acceptable as boosters (please note the dose of the Moderna booster differs from the primary-series dose).
		    See CDC recommendations for changing guidance on boosters.
		• Viral vector vaccine: Johnson & Johnson's Janssen Viral Vector COVID-19 Vaccine (JNJ-78436735)
		  ○ One-dose 0.5 mL IM with booster dose at least two months after first dose.
		  ○ FDA emergency use authorization for the Jansen vaccine is for ≥18 years of age; booster at least two months after first shot.
		  ○ Any of the COVID-19 vaccines in the US are approved as booster doses. ***See CDC recommendations for changing guidance on boosters.***

5	TETANUS-CONTAINING VACCINATIONS	Consider for all patients who do not have documentation of at least one dose within the last 10 years. • Indicated for adults every 10 years following final pediatric dose at 11 to 12 years. Adults should receive a single dose of Tdap then Td every 10 years, with all adults receiving at least one dose of Tdap.

Created & updated by the APhA-APPM Immunizing Pharmacists Special Interest Group (SIG).

Travel Immunization and Travel Health Card—
TRAVEL-SPECIFIC VACCINES

For a complete list by country go the CDC website.

VACCINE	INDICATION OR WHEN TO CONSIDER USING & DESCRIPTION
1 CHOLERA VACCINE	Vaxchora® (lyophilized CVD 103-HgR): Consider only for adult patients from the United States going to areas of active cholera transmission. Is an oral, live-attenuated vaccine. • Active cholera transmission is defined as an area within a country with endemic or epidemic cholera caused by *V. cholerae* O1 & has had activity within the last year. Does not include areas of rare imported or sporadic cases. • Approved for persons 2 to 64 years of age. Single dose must be administered 10 days prior to potential exposure. • No data exists on safety and efficacy in pregnant or breast™stfeeding women and immunocompromised patients. • Not recommended for travelers not visiting areas of active cholera transmission. Pregnant women and clinicians must consider risks associated with travel to active cholera area. • Should not be given to patients who have taken antibiotics (oral or parenteral) in preceding 14 days. • If chloroquine is indicated, chloroquine must be started ≥ 10 days after cholera vaccination. • Buffer of cholera vaccine may interfere with enteric-coated Ty21a vaccine. Taking first Ty21a dose > 8 hours after cholera vaccine might ↓ potential interference. • May shed virus in stool for ≥ 7 days, potentially may transmit to close contacts. • Requires special mixing (with supplied buffer) and consumed by patient within 15 minutes after reconstitution. Follow medical waste disposal procedures. • Patients must avoid eating or drinking 60 minutes before and after ingestion of cholera vaccine. • Vaccine efficacy has been established at three months after vaccination. Safety and efficacy beyond three months or need for booster doses has not been established.
2 DENGUE VACCINE	Dengvaxia® (Dengue tetravalent live vaccine) is FDA approved in the US for children (9 to 16 years of age) who live in areas where dengue is common (e.g., US territories of American Samoa, Puerto Rico, US Virgin Islands) and who have had laboratory-confirmed prior dengue virus infection. • As of June 2021, ACIP recommends three doses of Dengvaxia® administered 6 months apart at 0, 6 & 12 months in persons 9 to 16 years of age with a laboratory-confirmed prior dengue infection and living in endemic areas. • Protects against all serotypes of the dengue virus (1, 2, 3 & 4). • Should not be used in individuals who do not live in endemic areas and have not been previously infected by any dengue virus or if previous infection history is unknown. It increases risk for severe dengue disease if infected after with the virus. • Contraindicated in immunosuppressed persons. • Requires reconstitution with saline diluent. Swirl gently without removing the needle. Resulting suspension should be colorless with potential trace amounts of white/translucent particles. If vial contains more than trace particles, it should be discarded. After reconstitution, administer immediately or refrigerate at 2 to 8°C for no more than 30 minutes.

Created & updated by the APhA-APPM Immunizing Pharmacists Special Interest Group (SIG).

Travel Immunization and Travel Health Card—
TRAVEL-SPECIFIC VACCINES *(continued)*

For a complete list by country go the CDC website.

	VACCINE	INDICATION OR WHEN TO CONSIDER USING & DESCRIPTION
3	EBOLA VACCINE	Ervebo® (*Zaire ebolavirus* vaccine) is not commonly available in the USA. It can be made available for pre-exposure vaccination to eligible people by the Assistant Secretary of Preparedness. Eligibility categories are: • Ebola virus disease responders – individuals responding to an outbreak of *Zaire ebolavirus* • Laboratorians & support staff working at Biosafety Level 4 facilities who work with the replication component *Zaire ebolavirus* • Health-care personnel at federally designated Ebola Treatment Centers involved in the transport and care of patients known or suspected to be infected with *Zaire ebolavirus*
4	JAPANESE ENCEPHALITIS (JE) VACCINE	Ixiaro® (inactivated Japanese encephalitis vaccine) is for long-term and recurrent travelers who plan to spend ≥ 1 month in endemic areas (Asia & parts of Western Pacific) during JE virus transmission season or expatriates traveling to rural or agricultural areas during high-risk period of JE virus transmission. • May consider for short-term travelers (< 1 month) to endemic areas if: during JE virus transmission season/outside an urban area & activities will increase risk of JE virus exposure; traveling to area with ongoing JE outbreak or specific destination unknown or during peak transmission season (usually May to December, but may differ based on country, activities, or duration of travel.) • Not recommended for short-term travelers whose visits will be restricted to urban areas or times outside a well-defined JE virus transmission season. • The vaccination dose & primary schedule vary by age (*all age groups: complete two-dose series at least one week before potential exposure*): | 2 to 35 months	2 doses (0.25 mL ea.) IM on days 0 & 28	3 to 17 years	2 doses (0.5 mL ea.) IM on days 0 & 28 | |---|---|---|---| | 18 to 65 years | 2 doses (0.5 mL ea.) IM on days 0 & 7 to 28; only age group with accelerated schedule | > 65 years | 2 doses (0.5 mL ea.) IM on days 0 & 28 | • Booster dose should be administered ≥ 1 year after completion of primary series for those with continued exposure risk. Booster doses for children < 3 years = 0.25 mL & adults/children > 3 years = 0.5mL. Not data available for booster doses administered two years after primary series
5	RABIES VACCINE	Per CDC recommendations, consider pre-exposure vaccine Imovax Rabies® or RabAvert®: For those who plan to or may come in contact with potentially rabid animals (e.g., biologist, veterinarians, agriculture specialist, etc.) &/or with prolonged travel or shorter stays in high-risk areas (e.g., epidemic outbreaks) or with extensive outdoor stays in remote areas where medical care may be delayed or difficult. • Current recommendations for immunocompetent people are two of the 1 mL doses on days 0 and 7. • Pre-exposure vaccination simplifies post-exposure regimen but does not eliminate need for vaccination after exposure. Rabies vaccine should not be given if time does not permit completion of series prior to departure.

Created & updated by the APhA-APPM Immunizing Pharmacists Special Interest Group (SIG)

Travel Immunization and Travel Health Card—
TRAVEL-SPECIFIC VACCINES *(continued)*

For a complete list by country go the CDC website.

	VACCINE	INDICATION OR WHEN TO CONSIDER USING & DESCRIPTION

6	**TYPHOID VACCINE**	For all persons traveling to increased risk areas of exposure to Salmonella Typhi. Formulation choice based on age, patient preference, and departure time.
		• Typhim Vi® (ViCPS, Sanofi Pasteur): Inactivated polysaccharide vaccine approved for patients ages ≥ 2 as a single IM dose administered ≥ 2 weeks prior to possible exposure for optimal protection but may be used for last-minute travelers. Dosed every two years if at continued risk.
		• Vivotif® (Ty21a, Emergent Bio Solutions): Live-attenuated oral vaccine approved for patients ages ≥ 6 taken as one capsule every other day one hour before a meal with cold or lukewarm drink for a total of four days. The regimen should be completed one week prior to possible exposure. Refrigerate capsules. May be re-dosed every five years if continued risk.
		  ○ Avoid combination with antibiotics. Delay vaccine series until > 3 days after antibiotic course is complete or complete series > 7 days before first antibiotic dose.
		  ○ Antimalarial agents (e.g., mefloquine, chloroquine, atovaquone/proguanil, and pyrimethamine/sulfadoxine), when used at prophylaxis doses, may be administered at the same time as the vaccine. Manufacturer recommendations state to administer at least three days after last vaccine dose.
		  ○ Avoid in pregnancy by using contraception for four weeks after vaccine in female patients with childbearing potential.
		  ○ If oral vaccine is not available due to ongoing production or supply issues, the injectable vaccine can be used.

7	**YELLOW FEVER VACCINE**	Consider use in those who are traveling to or through yellow fever endemic areas or when proof of vaccination is required for entry. Consult the CDC for destination-specific recommendations. • Yellow fever vaccine should be avoided in children < 6 months, those allergic to gelatin, latex, or egg proteins, or in those who are severely immunocompromised. HIV infection with CD4 count 200 to 499/mm³ is a precaution for yellow fever vaccine. May offer waiver instead of vaccination when benefit does not outweigh risk. • Consider risk-benefit, especially in children 6 to 8 months and patients ≥ 60 years old who have never previously received the vaccine. • Women who are pregnant should only be vaccinated if travel to an endemic area is unavoidable and benefit of vaccination outweighs risk. • WHO/CDC now considers a single dose to be protective for life. Country-specific regulations may still require revaccination every 10 years and require initial administration ***at least 10 days before travel*** • ***Due to a current vaccine shortage in the US, patients may need to locate yellow fever vaccination clinics on the CDC website***
8	**MALARIA VACCINE**	The WHO formally recommended Mosquirix® (RTS, S/AS01) malaria vaccine for expanded use among children in sub-Saharan Africa and other regions with moderate to high malaria transmission beginning October 2021. ***Children ≥ 5 months should receive a schedule of four doses with first three doses given at least one month apart for each dose, and a fourth dose 15 to 18 months after the third dose.*** This is the first vaccine recommended to combat malaria.

Sample References:
- Advisory Committee on Immunization Practices (ACIP): Vaccines for Children Program Vaccines to Prevent Hepatitis A. Resolution No. 6/19-6. Adopted June 2019.
- Centers for Disease Control & Prevention (CDC). CDC Health Info for International Travel 2020. Oxford University Press, 2019.
- CDC. Recommended Adult Immunization Schedule by Medical Condition & Other Indications, US, 2020.
- CDC. COVID-19. Last reviewed 2021.
- Jackson BR, Iqbal S, Mahon B. Updated Recommendations for the Use of Typhoid Vaccine. ACIP, US, 2015. *MMWR Mortal Wkly Rep* 2015; 64(11): 305–8.
- Schillie S, Vellozzi C, Reingold A, et al. Prevention of Hepatitis B Virus Infection in the United States. Recommendations of ACIP for Use of Hepatitis B Vaccine with a Novel Adjuvant. *MMWR Morb Mortal Wkly Rep* 2018; 67: 455–8.

Travel Immunization and Travel Health Card—
NON-VACCINE TRAVEL CONSIDERATIONS

For a complete list of vaccinations recommended by country go the CDC Traveler's Health website.

	VACCINE	INDICATION OR WHEN TO CONSIDER USING & DESCRIPTION
1	TUBERCULOSIS (TB) TESTING	Only for patients at increased risk of exposure during travel, including health-care workers, those who will have contact with prison or homeless populations, and expatriates to countries with high TB prevalence. • Two-step tuberculin skin testing (TST) should be given prior to travel (second test 1 to 3 weeks after first) with repeat testing every 6 to 12 months during possible exposure period and 8 to 12 weeks after return. • Alternative test: interferon-gamma release assays (IGRA) is more specific in patients who have received BCG vaccines) may also be used if time before departure is too short for two-step TST. • TST may also be considered for VFR patients to document status prior to travel, which can aid in interpretation of future positive tests.
2	MALARIA CHEMO-PROPHYLAXIS	Use mosquito avoidance and personal protective measures (i.e., insect repellent, long sleeves/pants, sleeping in mosquito-free setting, or using insecticide-treated bed net) for all travelers to areas where malaria transmission occurs. Assess itinerary to determine risk for exposure & other specific factors in choice of chemoprophylaxis regimen.

Resistance Considerations	Health Considerations
• When deciding on chemoprophylaxis regimen, consider drug resistance in areas of travel, length of travel, traveler's medical conditions, allergy history, concomitant medications, and potential side effects. • Chloroquine and primaquine usefulness is limited to Central America, as resistance exists in all other areas. • Avoid mefloquine in parts of Southeast Asia (e.g., Thailand) due to resistance.	• Avoid mefloquine with personal or family history of psychiatric diagnosis, including depression and anxiety. • Avoid mefloquine and tafenoquine in patients with personal or family history of psychiatric conditions. • Avoid primaquine and tafenoquine in patients who do not have documented normal G6PD levels due to risk of death due to hemolysis in deficient patients.

3	STAND-BY EMERGENCY SELF-TREATEMENT OF TRAVELER'S DIARRHEA (TD)	For all travelers to developing countries.
		• First-line antibiotics include ciprofloxacin, levofloxacin, and azithromycin.
		  ◦ Avoid fluoroquinolones with travel to SE Asia (resistant strains of *Campylobacter* prevalent (e.g., Thailand))
		  ◦ Antimotility agents (e.g., bismuth subsalicylate and loperamide) may be recommended as adjunct symptomatic therapy.
		• Prophylactic antibiotics not recommended except in high-risk travelers (e.g., immunocompromised). Consider alternate SBET antibiotics and prophylaxis in these patients.

4	ACETAZOLAMIDE ALTITUDE ILLNESS PROPHYLAXIS	For all travelers at moderate to high risk for altitude illness, including those planning rapid ascents of > 1,600 ft (sleeping altitude) above 9,800ft with/without extra acclimatization days every 3,300 ft or those with history of altitude illness. • Usual dosing: 125 mg (or 250 mg if >100 kg) twice daily beginning one day prior to ascent, during ascent, and for two days at destination altitude.

Created & updated by the APhA-APPM Immunizing Pharmacists Special Interest Group (SIG).

Conversions

Pounds to Kilograms

lb	=	kg	lb	=	kg	lb	=	kg
1		0.45	70		31.75	140		63.50
5		2.27	75		34.02	145		65.77
10		4.54	80		36.29	150		68.04
15		6.80	85		38.56	155		70.31
20		9.07	90		40.82	160		72.58
25		11.34	95		43.09	165		74.84
30		13.61	100		45.36	170		77.11
35		15.88	105		47.63	175		79.38
40		18.14	110		49.90	180		81.65
45		20.41	115		52.16	185		83.92
50		22.68	120		54.43	190		86.18
55		24.95	125		56.70	195		88.45
60		27.22	130		58.91	200		90.72
65		29.48	135		61.24			

Temperature

Fahrenheit to Centigrade or Celsius: (°F − 32) × 5/9 = °C
Centigrade or Celsius to Fahrenheit: (°C × 9/5) + 32 = °F

°C	=	°F	°C	=	°F	°C	=	°F
100.0		212.0	39.0		102.2	36.8		98.2
50.0		122.0	38.8		101.8	36.6		97.9
41.0		105.8	38.6		101.5	36.4		97.5
40.8		105.4	38.4		101.1	36.2		97.2
40.6		105.1	38.2		100.8	36.0		96.8
40.4		104.7	38.0		100.4	35.8		96.4
40.2		104.4	37.8		100.1	35.6		96.1
40.0		104.0	37.6		99.7	35.4		95.7
39.8		103.6	37.4		99.3	35.2		95.4
39.6		103.3	37.2		99.0	35.5		95.0
39.4		102.9	37.0		98.6	0		32.0
39.2		102.6						

Weights and Measures

Category	Unit	Conversion
Exact Equivalents	1 ounce (oz)	28.35 grams (g)
	1 pound (lb)	453.6 g (0.4536 kilograms [kg])
	1 fluid oz (fl oz)	29.57 mL
	1 pint (pt)	473.2 mL
	1 quart (qt)	946.4 mL
Metric Conversions	1 kg	1000 g
	1 g	1000 mg
	1 mg	1000 µg
Approximate Measures: Liquids	1 fl oz	30 mL
	1 cup (8 fl oz)	240 mL
	1 pint (16 fl oz)	480 mL
	1 quart (32 fl oz)	960 mL
	1 gallon (128 fl oz)	3800 mL
Approximate Measures: Weights	1 oz	30 g
	1 lb (16 oz)	480 g
	15 grains	1 g
	1 grain	60 mg

Apothecary Equivalents

Category	Unit	Conversion
Weight	1 scruple	20 grains
	60 grains	1 dram
	8 drams	1 ounce
	1 ounce	480 grains
	16 ounces	1 pound (lb)
	1 g	15.43 grains (gr)
	1 gr	64.8 mg
	1 mg	1/65 gr
	0.8 mg	1/80 gr
	0.6 mg	1/100 gr
	0.5 mg	1/120 gr
	0.4 mg	1/150 gr
	0.3 mg	1/200 gr
	0.2 mg	1/300 gr
	0.12 mg	1/500 gr
	0.1 mg	1/600 gr
Volume	60 minims	1 fluidram
	8 fluidrams	1 fluid ounce
	1 fluid once	480 minims
	16 fluid ounces	1 pint (pt)
	1 mL	16.23 minims
	1 minim	0.06 mL

Opioid Conversions

Equianalgesic Dosing

Opioid Agonist	Oral Dose (PO)	Parenteral Dose (IV, SC, IM)	Duration of Action (h)
Morphine (IR)	30 mg	10 mg	3 to 4
HYDROmorphone	7.5 mg	1.5 mg	3 to 4
OXYcodone	20 mg	---	3 to 4
HYDROcodone	30 mg	---	3 to 4
OXYmorphone	10 mg	1 mg	3 to 4
Codeine	200 mg	100 mg	4
Fentanyl	---	0.1 mg	2

Note: In use of this table, please consider the following limitations:
1. *Limitation to studies that established equianalgesic dosing: Dosing based on studies using opioid doses in acute, short-term use. Chronic use requirements may differ for patients. Mean values were often with large variability in potency in study participants. Studies also were based on single dose studies.*
2. *Switching doses may require reducing the dosage of the new agent by 25 to 50% (% may vary). See table below on "Guidance for Changing Opioid Therapy." Titrate doses to avoid incidence of side effects, particularly with high doses. Monitor patients closely.*
3. *This chart should be used as a guide only. Consider patient-specific factors, such as age, body surface area, organ dysfunction, drug tolerance, type of pain (neuropathic or nociceptive; persistent vs. intermittent; chronic vs. acute), pharmacogenetics, drug–drug interactions, and drug–food interactions when selecting dosing for patients.*
4. *Conversion risks may exist for patients particularly (e.g., buprenorphine; methadone).*
5. *Some dosing equivalencies may not be bidirectional.*
6. *Note that this conversion table is not for transdermal (TD) fentanyl. 1 mcg/hour of TD fentanyl is ~ equivalent to 2 mg per day of oral (PO) morphine.*
IR = immediate release.

References:
https://rsds.org/wp-content/uploads/2014/12/MEDD-White-Paper-FINAL.pdf
https://www.jpsmjournal.com/article/S0885-3924(09)00630-7/fulltext
Breitbart W, Chandler S, Ellison N, Enck RE, Lefkowitz M, Payne R. An alternative algorithm for dosing transdermal fentanyl for cancer-related pain. Palliative and Supportive Care. 2000 May 1;14(5). https://www.cancernetwork.com/palliative-and-supportive-care/alternative-algorithm-dosing-transdermal-fentanyl-cancer-related-pain/page/0/1 (Accessed 2021)

Guidance for Changing Opioid Therapy

Step	Description
1	Determine the total 24-hour dose of the currently prescribed analgesic.
2	Convert the currently prescribed opioid to an equivalent dose of the desired opioid and formulation.
3	If pain is controlled, start at 50% to 75% of the equianalgesic dose to account for incomplete cross-tolerance between opioids. If pain is uncontrolled, then start at 100% of the dose.
4	Determine the strength per dose by dividing the dose calculated in Step 3 by the dosing interval. • Choose a dosing interval consistent with the medication duration of action of the new opioid/formulation.
5	Provide an appropriate "rescue" dose for breakthrough pain when applicable. • 10 to 15% of the total opioid dose given every 3 to 4 hours as needed.
6	Titrate baseline and as-needed dose to provide effective pain relief.
7	Use stimulant laxative (seena) or osmotic laxative (polyethylene glycol [PEG]) as constipation prophylaxis.

Monitoring for Respiratory Depression
• Unintended increased sedation from opioids is a sign that the patient may be at risk for respiratory depression.

Signs of Respiratory Depression
• Respiratory rate < 10 breaths per minute
• Paradoxic rhythm with little chest expansion
• Evidence of advancing sedation
• Poor respiratory effort or quality
• Snoring or noisy respirations
• Desaturation
• Cold or purple/blueish extremities
• ± pinpoint pupils

Prepared by Jessica Carswell; updated by Kashelle Lockman

Systemic Corticosteroid Conversions

Glucocorticoid	Approximate Equivalency	Potency Relative to Hydrocortisone		Half-life T½	Dosage Forms
		Anti-inflammatory	Mineral Corticoid		
Short Acting					
Cortisone	25 mg	0.8 mg	0.8 mg	8 to 12 hours	PO, IM
Hydrocortisone	20 mg	1 mg	1 mg		IV, IM, PO
Intermediate Acting					
Methylprednisolone	4 mg	5 mg	0.5 mg	12 to 36 hours	IV, IM, PO
Prednisolone	5 mg	4 mg	0.8 mg		IV, PO
Prednisone	5 mg	4 mg	0.8 mg		PO **ONLY**
Triamcinolone	4 mg	5 mg	0 mg		IM, PO
Long Acting					
Betamethasone	0.6 to 0.75 mg	20 to 30 mg	0	36 to 54 hours	IM, PO
Dexamethasone	0.75 mg	20 to 30 mg	0	36 to 72 hours	IV, IM, PO

Note: PO = oral; IM = intramuscular; IV = intravenous.

Suggested References
- Lexi-Drugs: Corticosteroids Systemic Equivalencies, Drug Monographs
- Facts & Comparisons: Equivalencies, Potencies, & T½, Monographs
- Micromedex: Drug Monographs
- Asare K. Diagnosis & treatment of adrenal insufficiency in the critically ill patient. Pharmacotherapy. 2007 Nov;27(11):1512–28.
- Liu D, Ahmet A, Ward L, et al. A practical guide to the monitoring & management of the complications of systemic corticosteroid therapy. Allergy, Asthma, and Clinical Immunology. 2013. 1, 30.

Prepared by Jenna Blunt and Jeanine P. Abrons

How to Work Up a Patient (*Inpatient/Ambulatory Care*)

Steps:

1. **Collect information that is generally constant in the visit** (e.g., demographics, name, date of birth, etc.).
   a. Add it into this form — Side 1:
      i. Name, age, gender identity, date of birth (DOB), date (or date of admission), chief complaint or reason for seeking care, history of present illness (HPI), past medical history (PMH), social history (SH), and chronic problem list.
2. **Collect information that you may need to see variable trends** (e.g., laboratory values).
   a. Add it into this form — Side 1:
      i. Current weight, height, temperature, blood pressure, heart rate, respiration rate, O2, CMP and CBC (inpatient) etc.
3. **Conduct calculations.**
   a. Ideal Body Weight (IBW)

Calculation	Sex/Notes	Calculation
Ideal Body Weight (IBW) (in kg)	Male	50 + (2.3 x height in inches over 5 feet)
	Female	45.5 + (2.3 x height in inches over 5 feet)
	Boys ≥ 5 feet tall	39 + (2.27 x height in inches over 5 feet)
	Girls ≥ 5 feet tall	42.2 + (2.27 x height in inches over 5 feet)
	Boys & Girls < 5 feet tall	(Height^2 x 1.65)/1000

Body Mass Index (BMI)

Calculation	Gender/Notes	Calculation
Body Surface Area (BSA) (in m^2)	All	• Mosteller:[1] $\sqrt{([\text{height (cm)} \times \text{weight (kg)}] / 3600)}$ • Lam:[2] $\sqrt{([\text{height (in)} \times \text{weight (lb)}] / 3131)}$ • DuBois & DuBois:[3] 0.007184 x height (cm)$^{0.725}$ x weight (kg)$^{0.425}$
Body Mass Index (in kg/m^2)	All/metric	• Weight (kg) / [height (m)]^2
	All/imperial	• Weight (lb) x 703 / height squared in (in^2)
Adjusted Body Weight		• (AjBW) = IBW + 0.4(ABW − IBW)

References
1. Mosteller RD. Simplified calculation of body-surface area [letter]. N Engl J Med. 1987;317(17):1098.
2. Lam TK, Leung DT. More on simplified calculation of body surface area [letter]. N Engl J Med. 1988;318(17):1130.
3. DuBois D, DuBois EF. A formula to estimate the approximate surface area if height and weight be known. Arch Int Med. 1916;17:863–71.

How to Work Up a Patient
(*Inpatient/Ambulatory Care*) (continued)

4. **Review Values** — Determine what is normal or abnormal.
   a. Normal Laboratory Values[a]
   b. Put up arrows = elevated labs; down arrows = low labs; dash = steady labs; circle new or important info; star = renally cleared values; ** = hepatically cleared drugs; + for new medications

Chemistries

Sodium	Chloride	Blood urea nitrogen (BUN)	Glucose (fasting)
135 to 146 mEq/L	95 to 108 mEq/L	7 to 30 mg/dL	$\leq$ 100 mg/dL
Potassium	Bicarbonate	Creatinine	
3.5 to 5.3 mEq/L	22 to 29 mEq/L	0.5 to 1.5 mg/dL	

Hematology

White blood cells
3.8 to 10.8 × 10³/µL

Hemoglobin
13.8 to 17.2 g/dL (men)
12 to 15.6 g/dL (women)

Hematocrit
41 to 50% (men)
35 to 46% (women)

Platelets
130 to 400 × 10³/µL

Test	Component	Normal Range
White Blood Cell (WBC) Differential	Bands	3 to 5%
	Basophils	0 to 1%
	Eosinophils	1 to 3%
	Lymphocytes	23 to 33%
	Monocytes	3 to 7%
	Neutrophils	57 to 67%
	Segmented neutrophils (segs)	54 to 62%
Red Blood Cell Count	Red blood cell count (men)	4.4 to 5.8 × 10⁶/µL
	Red blood cell count (women)	3.9 to 5.2 × 10⁶/µL
MCV	Mean corpuscular volume (MCV)	78 to 102 fL
MCH	Mean corpuscular hemoglobin (MCH)	27 to 33 pg/cell
MCHC	Mean corpuscular hemoglobin concentration (MCHC)	33 to 36%
Reticulocytes	Reticulocytes	0.5 to 2.3%
Arterial Blood Gases	Base excess	±2 mEq/L
	Bicarbonate (HCO₃)	22 to 26 mEq/L
	Oxygen saturation	94 to 100%
	Partial pressure of carbon dioxide ($PaCO_2$)	35 to 45 mmHg
	Partial pressure of oxygen (PaO_2)	75 to 100 mmHg
	pH	7.35 to 7.45

How to Work Up a Patient
(*Inpatient/Ambulatory Care*) *(continued)*

Review and Compare Patient Labs to Normal Laboratory Values[a] *(continued)*

Test	Component	Normal Range
Comprehensive Metabolic Panel	Albumin	3.5 to 5 g/dL
	Alkaline phosphatase (ALP)	20 to 125 U/L
	Bilirubin (Total)	≤ 1.3 mg/dL
See Chemistries figure for additional components	Bilirubin (Direct)	≤ 0.4 mg/dL
	Calcium (Total)	8.5 to 10.3 mg/dL
	Calcium (Ionized)	4.65 to 5.28 mg/dL
	Carbon dioxide	20 to 32 mEq/L
	Total serum protein	6.0 to 8.5 g/dL
Renal Function Panel*	Phosphorus	2.5 to 4.5 mg/dL
Uric Acid	Uric acid (men)	4.0 to 8.5 mg/dL
Enzymes	Alanine aminotransferase (ALT)	≤ 48 U/L
	Amylase	30 to 170 U/L
	Aspartate aminotransferase (AST)	≤ 42 U/L
	Creatine kinase (CK) (men)	≤ 235 U/L
	Creatine kinase (women)	≤ 190 U/L
	Gamma glutamyltransferase (GGT) (men)	≤ 65 U/L
	GGT (women)	≤ 45 U/L
	Lactic acid dehydrogenase (LD or LDH)	≤ 270 U/L
	Lipase	7 to 60 u/L

a. *Values given are for adults. Note that normal laboratory values vary widely between hospitals and laboratories; be sure to check the normal values at your site or institution.*

* *See also glucose; BUN; BUN/creatinine ratio; calcium; sodium; potassium; chloride; CO_2; albumin*

Calculate Fluid Composition and Perform Other Calculations

Patient Monitoring Calculations	
Monitoring Component	**Values/Description**
Serum Osmolality	mOsm/L = (2 x [Na^+]) + ([glucose in mg/dL]/18) + (BUN/2.8)
Anion Gap (AGE)	Na^+ − (Cl^- + HCO_3^-)
Water Deficit	0.6 x body weight (kg) x [1 − (140/Na^+)]
Free Water Deficit (FWD)	Normal total body weight (TBW) − Current TBW
	Normal TBW (Males) = Lean body weight (kg) x 0.6 L/kg
	Normal TBW (Females) = Lean body weight (kg) x 0.5 L/kg
	Current TBW = Normal TBW (140/Current [Na^+])
Corrected Sodium	$Na^+_{measured}$ + [((Serum glucose − 100)/100) x 1.6]
Corrected Calcium (based on albumin level)	[(normal albumin − patient's albumin) x 0.8] + patient's measured total Ca^{2+}
Chloride Deficit	0.4 x weight (kg) x (100 − $Cl^-_{measured}$)
Bicarbonate Deficit	(0.5 x kg) x (24 − $HCO^-_{3\,measured}$)

Note: BUN = blood urea nitrogen.

How to Work Up a Patient
(*Inpatient/Ambulatory Care*) *(continued)*

Consider Fluid Composition and Related Calculations *(continued)*

| Composition of Intravenous Fluids Used for Volume Resuscitation |||||
Fluid Type/Fluid Component	Sodium [Na+] in mEq/L	Chloride (Cl-) in mEq/L	mOsm/L	Other
Normal Saline (0.9% NS)	154	154	308	Isotonic
5% Dextrose/0.9% NS	154	154	560	Glucose: 50 g/L
Lactated Ringers (LR)	130	109	273	Potassium: K+ Calcium (Ca^{2+}) Lactate[1]
Dextrose 5% (5% D)	0	0	253	Glucose: 50 g/L
0.45% Normal Saline (1/2 NS)	77	77	154	
Dextrose 5%/0.45% NS	77	77	406	Glucose: 50 g/L

[1] K+: 4mEq/L; Ca^{2+}: 1.5 mEq/L; Lactate: 28 mEq/L; Modified based on information from Merck Manual—Emergency Medicine and Critical Care–Fluid Therapy.

Compare Patient Values with Electrolytes and Minerals

Laboratory Parameter	Normal Value
Sodium (Na+)	135 to 145 mEq/L
Potassium (K+)	3.5 to 5 mEq/L
Calcium (Ca^{2+})	8.5 to 10.5 mg/dL
Magnesium (Mg)	1.5 to 2.9 mEq/L
Phosphorus	3.7 to 4.5 mg/dL
Chloride (Cl-)	95 to 107 mEq/L
Bicarbonate (HCO_3^-)	22 to 28 mEq/L
Carbon Dioxide (CO_2)	24 to 32
Common Laboratory Parameters	
Blood Urea Nitrogen (BUN)	10 to 20
Serum Creatinine (SCr)	0.5 to 1 mg/dL
Glucose	65 to 99 mg/dL
White Blood Cells (WBC)	3.7 to 10.5 x 10^3/μL
Hemoglobin (Hgb)	11.9 to 15.5 g/dL
Hematocrit (Hct)	35 to 47%
Platelets	150 to 400 x 10^3/μL
Partial Thrombin Time (PTT)	23 to 31 seconds
Prothrombin Time (PT)	9 to 12 seconds
International Normalized Ratio (INR)	0.9 to 1.1

Note: ranges may vary based on institution-specific laboratory parameters.

How to Work Up a Patient
(*Inpatient/Ambulatory Care*) *(continued)*

5. **Propose potential differential diagnoses.**
   a. Match abnormal values and history of present illness to common medical diagnoses and medications.
6. **Review medications.**
   a. Match medications to an indication and assess status.
   b. Review appropriateness of drug, dose, frequency, route, renal/hepatic or weight/BSA-based adjustments for each indication.
   c. How is the medication being delivered?
   d. Assess for drug-drug and drug-disease interactions, risk categories (e.g., pregnancy, immunocompromised, age-based), and contraindications/black box warnings.
   e. Review safety.
   f. Review efficacy.
   g. Determine a reasonable follow-up frequency based on the setting and severity of the patient presentation.
7. **Create an acute and chronic problem list.**
   a. What problems can you and the pharmacy team solve?
   b. What problems do you need to bring up with the resident/healthcare provider or the interprofessional team?
   c. What things do you need to be clarified by the patient?
   d. Assess contributing causes of need to adjust patient's medications.
   e. Determine overlap between conditions (e.g., common symptoms that may create the potential for confusion of systems; drug/disease state interactions).
8. **Prioritize the problem list.**
   a. Determine what needs to be addressed first and subsequently.
      i. Consider medication and non-medication-related problems.
   b. Determine what would place the patient at increased risk for adverse effects or poor therapeutic outcomes (e.g., age, medications, genetics, clearance, the volume of distribution or potential for toxicity, etc.)
   c. Determine goals of therapy.
9. **Identify and create recommendations.**
   a. List acceptable medication changes or additions to address the prioritized problem list.
   b. Include drug, dose, route, frequency, frequency of monitoring/follow-up, and patient/provider education.
   c. Consider factors that would impact adherence or feasibility of regimen.
   d. Recommend needed immunizations based upon disease states, age, and other considerations.
   e. Identify opportunities for pharmacist-to-dose consults (per protocol).
10. **Review recommendations and double-check the process.**
    a. Consider social determinants of health.
    b. Consider social history.
    c. Consider the reliability of the information.
    d. Consider what could be missing.
    e. Consider untreated or insufficiently treated conditions.

References:
Lower Mainland Pharmacy Residency Program: Pharmacists' Workup of Drug Therapy (PWDT). http://www.lmpsresidency.com/residents/resident-manual/resident-resources. (Accessed October 2021)
McDonough RP. The pharmacist's 'patient work-up'. Pharmacy Today. 2017 Jul 1;23(7): 38.
May E. Erin May Pharm D. https://erinmayspharmd.com/life-as-a-resident/patient-workups-inpatient-medicine-rotations. (Accessed November 2021)
University of Minnesota. Pharmacotherapy Workup Plans. https://www.pharmacy.umn.edu/pharmacotherapy-workup-notes. (Accessed November 2021)

Sample Patient Workup Card for Use In Patient Care

Patient Information:

NAME		ROOM		PT #	
DATE		DOB		AGE/SEX	
HEIGHT		WEIGHT		IBW	
Pharmacy		Insurance			

Chief Complaint/ Reason for Seeking Care	Allergies/Sensitivities:

History of Present Illness (HPI):

Past Medical History (PMH):	Past Surgical History:

Social History (SH):

Caffeine		Alcohol	
Smoking		Drugs	
Occupation			
Exercise			
Dietary			

Chronic Problem List:

Problem List for Today:

Sample Patient Workup Card for Use in Patient Care *(continued)*

Vitals/Laboratory	Dates →						
Blood pressure (BP): *120/80 mmHg*							
Heart Rate: *60 to 90 bpm*							
RR: *12 to 20 bpm*							
Temperature (Max)							
O2 Saturation *80%*							
Pain Score							
In (mL)							
Out (mL)							
Net (mL)							
Electrolytes							
Na^{2+} *(135–145 mg/dL)*							
K^+ *(3.5–5 mg/dL)*							
Cl^- *(96–106 mg/dL)*							
HCO_3							
BUN *(10–24 mg/dL)*							
SCr *(0.5–1.3 mg/dL)*							
CrCl							
Glucose							
Ca^{2+} *(8.5–10.5)*							
Mg^{2+} *(1.6–2.7)*							
PO_4 *(2.5–4.5)*							
Liver							
Albumin *(3.4–4.7)*							
Alk Phos *(41–133)*							
AST *(7–26)*							
ALT *(3–23)*							
T.Bili *(0.1–1.2)*							
Coagulation							
INR *(0.9–1.2)*							
aPTT *(23–38 sec)*							
Hematology							
WBC *(4.5–11)*							
RBC *(4.5–5.0)*							
Hgb *(12–16)*							
Hct *(36–46)*							
MCV *(80–100)*							
MCH *(28–32)*							
MCHC *(31–35)*							
Platelets *(140–450)*							
Lymphocytes *(0.9–2.9)*							
Neutrophils *(1.8–6.8)*							
CRP *(< 6.3)*							

Document trends by using up, down, or neutral arrows.

Sample Patient Workup Card for Use in Patient Care *(continued)*

Date	Blood Glucose Values (mg/dL)/Times						
	12 am to 4 am	4 am to 8 am	8 am to 12 pm	12 pm to 4pm	4 pm to 8 pm	8 pm to 12 am	Notes/Insulin Used

Cultures

Date	Site	Result	Susceptible	Resistant

Imaging

Date	Site	Results/Notes

Medications

Antibiotics

Start	Antibiotic	Frequency/Start & Stop Dates	Indication

Intravenous Medications

Start	Medication	Route	Frequency	Notes/Timing

Sample Patient Workup Card for Use in Patient Care *(continued)*

Medications (continued)

As Needed Medications

Start	Medication	Route	Frequency	Notes/Timing

Scheduled Medications

Start	Medication	Route	Frequency	Notes/Timing

Medications Prior to Admission

Start	Medication	Route	Frequency	Notes/Timing

Other

Nutrition	
Social Work	
Resident/Med Student	

Other Notes

Acid and Base Imbalances—
An Overview and Implications for the Pharmacist

Acid–Base Imbalance	pH	PCO₂	HCO₃	Differential/Notes
Metabolic Acidosis	↓ Serum pH < 7.35	Normal or ↓	↓ HCO₃⁻ < 22mEq/L	• Related to ↑ acid • Signs & Symptoms (S&S): Headache; confusion; fruity breath; ↑ rate/depth of respirations (i.e., Kussmaul respiration → ↓CO₂, ↓ K⁺ [shifts into cells]); nausea; vomiting; dysrhythmias • Monitor: S&S; give NaHCO₃; supportive care for the underlying state • Diabetes; Addison's disease; Renal failure; ↑ acid production
Metabolic Alkalosis	↑ Serum pH > 7.45	Normal or ↑	↑ HCO₃⁻ > 26mEq/L	• Secondary to acid secretion loss (e.g., vomiting from upper gastrointestinal obstruction), thiazide & loop diuretics cause ↓ K⁺ to leave cells & H⁺ to enter; ↑ administration of HCO₃ • S&S: Paresthesia; tremors; shallow respirations → ↑ CO₂; dizziness; confusion; ↓ GI motility; ↓ K⁺ • Monitor: S&S; give NaCl; KCl & H₂ antagonists
Respiratory Acidosis	↓ Serum pH < 7.35	↑	Normal or ↑	• Retention from pulmonary edema, pneumonia, acute respiratory distress syndrome (ARDS), narcotic overdose, aspiration, emphysema, obstructed airway, or apnea • S&S: Shortness of breath (SOB); ↑ pulse; ↑ respirations; ↑ BP; restlessness; disorientation; ↑ K⁺; signs of intracranial pressure • Monitor: S&S; care for an underlying cause; mechanical ventilation
Respiratory Alkalosis	↑	↓ PaCO₂ > 42 mmHg	Normal or ↑	• Anemia; chronic heart failure; exuberant mechanical ventilation • S&S: ↑ pulse; ↓ K⁺; ↓ Ca²⁺; paresthesia; lightheadedness; dysrhythmias; ↓ LOC • Monitor: S&S; respirations; mechanical ventilator settings may have to ↓ rate &/or depth

ACLS Certification Institute. www.aclscertification.com

Prepared by Jeanine Abrons and Emily Paulus

Acid–Base Disorders—The Basics

- **Anion Gap:**
  Difference in electrical charge between the cations (positively charged ions) & the anions (negatively charged ions) in your blood
  - The number of positively and negatively charged molecules in your blood should equal a net charge of 0.
  - The anion gap is a calculation used to account for the unmeasured anions in your blood (e.g., sulfates, phosphates, blood proteins) that can be measured, but their electrical charge usually is not considered.
  - Calculation: Anion Gap = Sodium (Na^{2+}) − [Chloride (Cl^-) + Bicarbonate (HCO_3^-)]
    - Normal value = 12 mEq/L (Range of 8 to 16 mEq/L = acceptable)
- **How to Diagnose Acid–Base Disorders:**
  1. ***Step 1:*** Look at the pH (Determine the primary abnormality—acidosis or alkalosis).
  2. ***Step 2:*** Calculate the anion gap to determine the primary process (e.g., metabolic or respiratory).

Reference Range	Range
Reference Range if Calculation Employs Potassium	16 ± 4 mEq/L
Reference Range if Calculation Does Not Employ Potassium	12 ± 4 mEq/L
Type of Anion Gap	**Potential Causes Indicated**
↓ anion gap (< 6 mEq/L)	Hypoalbuminemia; plasma cell dyscrasia; monoclonal protein; bromide intoxication; normal variant
Normal anion gap (6 to 12 mEq/L)	HCO_3 loss (diarrhea); recovery from DKA; ileostomy fluid loss; carbonic anhydrase inhibitors; renal tubular acidosis; arginine/lysine; normal variant
↑ anion gap (> 12 mEq/L)	See MUDPILERS mnemonic under "Mnemonics for Acid–Base Disorders"

  3. ***Step 3:*** Consider if the cause is compensation vs. a concomitant primary process.
     a. Use calculations like Winter's formula for metabolic acidosis. Expected $PaCO_2 = 1.5(HCO_3) + (8 \pm 2)$
  4. ***Step 4:*** Calculate the excess anion gap and add it to the bicarbonate level (to further distinguish between acidosis and alkalosis). Look for the cause of the category.
     a. See mnemonics on Acid–Base Mnemonics Card.

- **How the body compensates:**
  - In respiratory disorders, the metabolic system compensates.
    - It happens in about 3 to 5 days—a slower system.
  - In metabolic disorders, the respiratory system compensates.
    - It happens in minutes to hours—a fast system.
    - Examples: Respiratory acidosis: body raises the HCO_3; Metabolic acidosis: body decreases CO_2

Prepared by Jeanine Abrons and Emily Paulus

Acid–Base Disorders—The Basics (continued)

Mnemonics for Acid–Base Disorders

Mnemonic	Description
MUDPILERS *For High–Anion Gap Metabolic Acidosis*	**M**ethanol or metformin; **U**remia; **D**iabetic ketoacidosis; **P**ropylene glycol; **I**soniazid, inborn error, or inhalants; **L**actic acidosis; **E**thylene glycol; **R**enal failure; **S**alicylates
HARDUP *For Non–Anion Gap Metabolic Acidosis*	**H**yperalimentation (e.g., starting TPN); **A**cetazolamide use; **R**enal tubular acidosis; **D**iarrhea; **U**retosigmoid fistula (due to HCO_3 wasting); **P**ancreatic fistula (due to alkali loss, the pancreas secretes HCO_3-rich fluid)
CLEVER PD *For Metabolic Alkalosis*	**C**ontraction (due to blood loss); **L**icorice; **E**ndocrine (Conn's/Cushing's/Batter's); **V**omiting/nasogastric suction; **E**xcess alkali; **R**efeeding alkalosis; **P**ost-hypercapnia; **D**iuretics
CANS *For Respiratory Acidosis*	**C**NS depression; **A**irway obstruction; **N**euromuscular disorders; **S**evere pneumonia, embolism, edema (pulmonary)
CHAMPS *For Respiratory Alkalosis*	**C**NS stimulation; **H**ypoxia; **A**nxiety; **M**echanical ventilation; **P**rogesterone; **S**alicylates or Sepsis
GOLDMARK *For Anion–Gap Metabolic Acidosis*	**G**lycols; **O**xoproline; **L**-lactate; **D**-lactate; **M**ethanol; **A**spirin; **R**enal failure; **K**etoacidosis (diabetic or alcoholic)

References:
International Emergency Medicine Project. https://iem-student.org/acid-base-disturbance/. Accessed November 2021; Dyson B. Acid-Base Disorders: Essentials for Pharmacists. https://www.tldrpharmacy.com/content/acid-base-disorders-essentials-for-pharmacists. Accessed November 2021; Wargo KA. ABCs of ABGs: A guide to interpreting acid-base disorders. Hospital Pharmacy. 2008 43(10):808–15; Metha AN, Emmett JB, Emmett M. GOLD MARK: an anion gap mnemonic for the 21st century. Lancet. 2008; 372(9642):892. doi:10.1016/S0140-6736(08)61398-7. PMID: 18790311.

Prepared by Jeanine Abrons and Emily Paulus

Creatinine Clearance Calculations

Name of Calculation	Formula	Appropriate Use
Cockcroft-Gault[1]	**Women:** $= \dfrac{[(140 - \text{age}) \times \text{weight (in kilograms [kg])}]}{72 \times [\text{serum creatinine in mg/dL}]} \times 0.85$ **Men:** $= \dfrac{[(140 - \text{age}) \times \text{weight (in kilograms [kg])}]}{72 \times [\text{serum creatinine in mg/dL}]}$	• Used frequently for medication dosing • *Note:* which weight to use in the calculation is based upon the specific drug (ideal, adjusted, or actual body weight) ○ This may require calling the company & may not be in package information. • While serum creatinine may be underestimated in frail or elderly patients, it may be overestimated in muscular patients.
Schwartz[2]	$= \dfrac{[\text{length in (cm)} \times k]}{\text{serum creatinine in mg/dL}}$ | Age/Classification	k value to use
---	---
1 to 52 weeks old	0.45
1 to 13 years old	0.55
Females: 13 to 18 years old	0.55
Males: 13 to 18 years old	0.7		• Used frequently in pediatric patients • Presents results as mL/minute/1.73m^2
MDRD (Modified Diet in Renal Disease)	Glomerular Filtration Rate: $= 175 \times \text{SCr}^{-1.154} \times \text{age}^{-0.203}$ $\times\ 1.212$ (if patient is black) $\times\ 0.742$ (if patient is female)	Used frequently in the staging of patients Not used for acute renal failure While serum creatinine may be underestimated in frail or elderly patients, it may be overestimated in muscular patients.

Recommended Resources/References
1. Cockcroft DW, Gault MH. Prediction of creatinine clearance from serum creatinine. Nephron. 1976;16(1):31–41.
2. Schwartz GJ, Haycock GB, Edelmann CM, Spitzer A. A simple estimate of glomerular filtration rate in children derived from body length and plasma creatinine. Pediatrics. 1976. 58:259–263.
3. Levey AS, Stevens LA, Schmid CH, Zhang YL et al. A new equation to estimate glomerular filtration rate. Ann Intern Med. 2009;150(9):604–12.

Prepared by Jessica Carswell; updated by Kashelle Lockman and Jeanine Abrons

Target Serum Concentrations for Selected Drugs

Reported ranges vary according to source. Ranges reported here are for reference purposes only. Decisions regarding treatment or management of patients should be based on reference intervals reported by the specific laboratory that performs the test. Target ranges represent those for an adult population.

Drug	Target Range
Carbamazepine	4 to 12 µg/mL
Chloramphenicol	10 to 20 µg/mL (peak) 5 to 10 µg/mL (trough) *Note: Levels represent targets for other infections; different targets exist for meningitis*
Cyclosporine	100 to 400 µg/mL (blood)
Digoxin	Heart Failure Therapeutic: 0.5 to 0.8 ng/mL Toxic: levels > 2ng/mL *Note: Levels should be drawn at least 6 to 8 hours after last dose, regardless of route of administration. Specific criteria exist on when to obtain concentration if loading dose is or is not given.*
Ethosuximide	40 to 100 µg/mL[a]
Lidocaine	Therapeutic: 1.5 to 5 µg/mL Toxic: > 6 µg/mL
Lithium	Therapeutic: 0.6 to 1.2 mEq/L Toxic: > 1.5 mEq/L *Note: Different targets exist for acute mania; prevention of episodes in patients with bipolar disorder & elderly patients.*
Phenobarbital	Infants/Children–Therapeutic: 10 to 40 mcg/mL Adults–Therapeutic: 10 to 40 µg/mL Toxic: > 40 µg/mL
Phenytoin	10 to 20 µg/mL[a]
Primidone	5 to 12 µg/mL[a]
Procainamide/ N-acetylprocainamide (NAPA)	Therapeutic: Procainamide: 4 to 10 mcg/mL; NAPA: 15 to 25 mcg/mL Combined: 10 to 30 mcg/mL
Quinidine	2 to 5 µg/mL[a]
Theophylline	10 to 20 µg/mL[a]
Valproic acid	50 to 100 µg/mL

a. Trough levels just prior to next dose.

Psychiatry Guidelines

Topic Area/ Associated Guideline	Publication/Website	Notes
Major Depressive Disorder	American Psychiatric Association (APA). Practice guideline for the treatment of patients with major depressive disorder. 3rd ed. Arlington (VA): American Psychiatric Association (APA); 2010; http://psychiatryonline.org/pb/assets/raw/sitewide/practiceguidelines/guidelines/mdd.pdf	Legacy practice guideline Updated in 2010
Obsessive-Compulsive Disorder	American Psychiatric Association (APA). Practice guideline for the treatment of patients with obsessive-compulsive disorder. Arlington (VA): American Psychiatric Association (APA); 2007; http://psychiatryonline.org/pb/assets/raw/sitewide/practice_guidelines/guidelines/ocd.pdf	Legacy practice guideline Updated in 2007 (Guideline watch in 2013)
Generalized Anxiety Disorders	National Collaborating Centre for Mental Health, National Collaborating Centre for Primary Care. Generalized anxiety disorder and panic disorder (with or without agoraphobia) in adults. Management in primary, secondary, and community care. London (UK): National Institute for Health and Clinical Excellence (NICE); 2011 Jan. 56 p. (Clinical guideline; no. 11) https://www.nice.org.uk/guidance/cg113	Legacy practice guideline Updated in 2011
Panic Disorder	APA. Practice guideline for the treatment of patients with panic disorder. 2nd ed. 2009; http://psychiatryonline.org/pb/assets/raw/sitewide/practice_guidelines/guidelines/panicdisorder.pdf	Legacy practice guideline Updated in 2009
Schizophrenia	APA. 2020 Guidelines for Treating Patients with Schizophrenia	Updated in 2020
Bipolar Disorder	APA. Practice guideline for the treatment of patients with bipolar disorder. http://psychiatryonline.org/pb/assets/raw/sitewide/practice_guidelines/guidelines/bipolar.pdf	Legacy practice guideline Updated in 2002 (Guideline watch 2005)
Substance Use Disorders	APA. Practice guideline for the treatment of patients with substance use disorders. 2nd ed. 2006; https://psychiatryonline.org/pb/assets/raw/sitewide/practice_guidelines/guidelines/substanceuse.pdf	Guideline watch 2007
Post-Traumatic Stress Disorder	VA/DOD. Clinical practice guideline for the management of posttraumatic stress disorder and acute stress disorder. 2017; https://www.healthquality.va.gov/guidelines/MH/ptsd/VADoDPTSDCPGFinal012418.pdf	

Resources for the Practicing Pharmacist

Resource	Website	Use for Pharmacy
Neuroscience Education Institute	http://neiglobal.com	Information regarding mental health pathophysiology and psychopharmacology; medication comparisons; clinical practice resources
College of Psychiatric & Neurologic Pharmacists	http://cpnp.org	Psychiatric-related job postings; residency information; board certification information; continuing education resources; suggested readings
American Psychiatric Association	http://www.psychiatry.org	Fact brochures; several psychiatry-related publications; continuing education resources; clinical practice resources
Stahl's Essential Psychopharmacology Online	https://stahlonline.cambridge.org	Index available by drug; covers the therapeutic use and mechanisms; guidance on how to select agents; drug interactions; dosing tips; teacher images for presentation

Prepared by Sara F. Dugan; updated with Benjamin Miskle

Psychiatric Medications

Medication Class	Common Adverse Drug Reactions	Clinical Pearls
Selective Serotonin Reuptake Inhibitors (SSRIs)	Somnolence; fatigue; insomnia; nausea; dry mouth; diaphoresis; sexual dysfunction; weakness (Fluoxetine); headache	• Commonly utilized for the treatment of depression or anxiety disorders. • Symptom improvement often takes weeks of therapy. • Drug interactions due to CYP inhibition occur with some medications in this class.
Serotonin-Norepinephrine Reuptake Inhibitors (SNRIs)	Fatigue; headache; nausea; dizziness; dry mouth; insomnia; decreased appetite; hyperhidrosis (Desvenlafaxine)	• Commonly utilized for the treatment of depression or anxiety disorders. • Symptom improvement often takes weeks of therapy. • Elevated blood pressure (BP) has been reported with some medications in this class.
Tricyclic Antidepressants (TCAs)	Weight gain; sexual dysfunction; hypotension; QT abnormalities; dry mouth; constipation; nausea; somnolence	• Commonly utilized for many conditions including depression & anxiety disorders. • Symptom improvement often takes weeks. • Tolerability & potential toxicity are a greater concern with this class of medications.
Benzodiazepines	Sedation; dizziness; drowsiness; unsteadiness; hypotension; weakness	• Commonly used for the treatment of agitation, anxiety, insomnia, or seizure disorders. • Improvement is seen relatively quickly. • Benzodiazepines have the potential to cause dependence. • Abrupt discontinuation may result in withdrawal seizures.
Second Generation Antipsychotics (SGA)	Sedation; dizziness; hypotension; weight gain; abnormal muscle movements; elevations in glucose or cholesterol levels	• Commonly used for the treatment of schizophrenia and bipolar disorder, may also be used as adjunct treatment of depression. • Monitoring for movement disorders is important to screen for & prevent the development of tardive dyskinesia. • Regular metabolic monitoring of BP, weight, glucose, & cholesterol levels is recommended.

Note: CYP = cyctochrome P450.

Prepared by Sara E. Dugan; updated by Ben Miskle

Nutrition

Harris–Benedict Equation for Basic Metabolic Rate

Male
- $66.47 + (13.7 \times kg) + (5 \times cm) - (6.7 \times years) = kcal/day$

Female
- $655.1 + (9.56 \times kg) + (1.85 \times cm) - (4.68 \times years) = kcal/day$

Notes
- ↑ metabolic requirements can be factored in by multiplying the kcal/day by an injury factor (between 1 & 2.5)

Ideal Body Weight Equation

Male
- $50\ kg + (2.3\ kg \times inch\ over\ 5\ ft)$

Female
- $45.5\ kg + (2.3\ kg \times inch\ over\ 5\ ft)$

Enteral Nutrition

Indications for Use "If the gut works, use it."	• Failed swallow evaluation • Esophageal mass • Intubation • Unable to meet oral (PO) intake needs • Functioning gastrointestinal (GI) tract
Sample Indications for Frequency (Duration) *Select option best for patient care*	**Continuous (24 hours)** • With initiation of enteral feeds • With labile blood sugars difficult to manage on cyclic/bolus feeds **Nocturnal or cyclic (12 to 16 hours)** • If tube feeds (TF) are used to supplement oral intake. • If TF tolerated at a higher rate: will allow more time away from feeding pump **Bolus (never an option with J-tubes)** • To simulate routine meal time schedule

Total Parenteral Nutrition (TPN)

Indications for Use	• Nonfunctioning GI tract • Necessity for bowel rest • GI obstruction • GI dysfunction/malabsorption • Significant GI resection
Calculating TPN	• Weight based • Access-site dependent (central vs. peripheral) 1. Determine macronutrients 2. Determine elepctrolytes (based on daily labs & predicted daily requirements) 3. Determine volume/fluid needs
Ordering TPN	• Reassess electrolytes & blood sugars daily • Monitor kidney function, volume status, & current patient presentation • Evaluate infusion rate rate – continuous infusion vs. cyclic infusion with ramp up/ramp down rates. Typical goal is to cycle parenteral nutrition when electrolytes and blood sugars tolerate.
Weaning TPN	• Continue TPN until > 60% of PO diet is tolerated • Obtain blood glucose 1 hour after TPN is discontinued • Many strategies for weaning can include a set ramp up/ramp down rate, or can be more flexible like a pre-specified rate reduction (reducing rate by 50% every 20 minutes over an hour)

Nutrition *(continued)*

Common Daily Requirements for Parenteral Nutrition

Component	Standard Requirement	Commonly Formulated within Parenteral Nutrition Solutions
Water	25 to 40 mL/kg	
Calcium	10 to 15 mEq	Calcium gluconate; calcium chloride
Magnesium	8 to 20 mEq	Magnesium sulfate; magnesium chloride
Phosphorus	20 to 40 mmol	Sodium phosphate; potassium phosphate
Potassium	1 to 2 mEq/kg	Potassium chloride; potassium acetate; potassium phosphate
Sodium	1 to 2 mEq/kg	Sodium chloride; sodium acetate; sodium phosphate
Acetate	As needed to maintain acid-base balance	Sodium acetate; potassium acetate
Chloride	As needed to maintain acid-base balance	Sodium chloride; potassium chloride; magnesium chloride; calcium chloride

Reference: Mirtallo J, Canada T, Johnson D, et al. Safe Practices for Parenteral Nutrition. *Journal of Parenteral and Enteral Nutrition, 6,* S39–70. 2004.

Miscellaneous Monitoring Associated with Total Parenteral Nutrition (TPN)

Consideration	Information
Albumin	3 weeks half-life
Prealbumin	2 day half-life
Complete metabolic panel (CMP) Complete blood counts (CBC)	Monitor daily during acute inpatient hospitalization. As patient stabilizes or goes home on TPN, labs can be done less frequently (twice weekly, weekly, or bi-weekly).
Lipid panel	Monitored frequently during acute inpatient hospitalization in patients receiving lipid emulsion therapy.
Vitamins, minerals	Check if a deficiency is suspected; otherwise consider yearly.
Central line infection	Patients should be educated on signs/symptoms of an infection in a central line so they can conduct daily surveillance (e.g., redness, tenderness, oozing, fever, chills, swelling, pain). If an infection is suspected, it is important that the patient seek medical attention in a timely fashion.

Sample References
1. Kreymann KG, Berger MM, Deutz NE, et al. ESPEN Guidelines on Enteral Nutrition: Intensive Care. Clin Nutrition. 2006;25(2):210–23.
2. Madsen H, Frankel EH. The Hitchhiker's Guide to Parenteral Nutrition Management for Adult Patients. Practical Gastroenterology. 2006;46–68.
3. Barnadas G. Navigating Home Care: Parenteral Nutrition – Part 2. Practical Gastroenterology, 2003. https://med.virginia.edu/ginutrition/wp-content/uploads/sites/199/2015/11/practicalgastro-nov03.pdf (Accessed 2021)

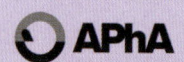

Nutrition *(continued)*

Calculating TPN

Step	Description of Step
1. Calculate Energy (Caloric) Needs	• Use the Harris-Benedict equation × activity × stress factor = energy (kcal), or you may use a scale. ○ The calories from protein, carbohydrates, & lipids should add up to this total.

Patient Description *Notes*	Energy Needs (Caloric) *Note: use actual body weight unless otherwise specified*
Well nourished, healthy, & requires maintenance therapy	• 20 to 25 kcal/kg
Critically ill; has metabolic stress; with recent trauma or is undernourished	• 25 to 30 kcal/kg
Critically ill & obese (BMI ≥ 30) • *Consider permissive underfeeding, hypocaloric high-protein feeding, or eucaloric feeding*	• **Using actual body weight:** 11 to 14 kcal/kg OR • **Using ideal body weight:** 22 to 25 kcal/kg
Acute renal failure or chronic kidney disease (CKD)	• 25 to 30 kcal/kg

Step	Description of Step
2. Determine Protein Needs	• High protein content may be more appropriate during the acute stages of critical illness • To calculate grams (g) of protein supplied in a solution, multiply total volume of amino acids (in mL) by the amino acid concentration. • Protein provides ~ 4 kcal/gram.

Patient Description *Notes*	Protein Requirements *Note: Use ideal body weight*
Well nourished, healthy, & requires maintenance therapy	• 0.8 to 1 g/kg
Critically ill; has metabolic stress; with recent trauma or is undernourished	• 1.2 to 2 g/kg
Critically ill & obese (BMI ≥ 30) • *Consider permissive underfeeding, hypocaloric high-protein feeding or eucaloric feeding*	• BMI of 30 to 40: 2 g/kg • BMI > 40: 2.5 g/kg
Acute renal failure or chronic kidney disease (CKD)	• Acute kidney injury (AKI) ± intermittent hemodialysis (iHD): 1.2 to 2 g/kg • CRRT: 2 to 2.5 g/kg • CKD Stage 3 or 4, not acutely ill: 0.3 to 0.6 g/kg • CKD Stage 5 with iHD 3 times per week: 1.2 g/kg • CKD Stage 5 with peritoneal dialysis daily: 1.3 g/kg

Nutrition *(continued)*

Step	Description of Step
3. Calculate the Fat (Lipids) Needed Based on Total Energy Needs	• Fat needs: 1 to 2.5 g of fat/kg or 15 to 30% of nonprotein kcal (maximum tolerance of 2.5 g/kg body weight & 60% of energy from fat) • Fat: 9 kcal/gram • Common caloric intake of available formulation: | Lipid Formulation	Kcal/mL
10% fat emulsion	1.1 kcal/mL
20% fat emulsion	2 kcal/mL
30% fat emulsion	3 kcal/mL	
4. Calculate the Carbohydrates (CHO)	• Determine needs by subtracting fat (lipid) needs & protein calorie needs from total energy (caloric) needs. Remaining amount is needed kcal from CHO. Take kcal CHO needed/kcal per 1 L of dextrose solution = mL dextrose solution needed. • Dextrose monohydrate = 3.4 kcal/g • Determine energy content of 1 L of formulate by multiplying mL x percentage of dextrose in dextrose solution. ○ Common formulations: dextrose 50% 1 L = 1,700 kcal; dextrose 70% 1 L = 2,380 kcal • Maximum rate of administration should not exceed 5 mg CHO/kg/min (could lead to hyperglycemia, liver dysfunction, & ↑ CO_2 production)
5. Calculate the Fluid Needs	• Fluid-restricted formulas with higher caloric density (kcal/mL) are available but may cause ↑ diarrhea due to ↑ osmolality • Fluid needs: 25 to 35 mL/kg/day × feeding weight (kg) = fluid needs/day (mL)
6. Determine Electrolyte Needs	Consider determining electrolyte formulations in the following order: (1) phosphate (sodium or potassium), (2) potassium (acetate or chloride), (3) sodium (acetate or chloride), (4) magnesium, & (5) calcium in order to take formulations into consideration efficiently.

7. Determine Vitamin, Mineral, & Additives	• Vitamin solutions include 12 vitamins.
	• Trace elements include copper, zinc, manganese, chromium, & selenium.
	  ○ Cholestasis: caution with manganese & copper—consider dose reduction or omission
	  ○ Renal dysfunction: caution with chromium use—consider reduction or omission
	• Other additives may include insulin, H2 receptor antagonists, & iron as examples.

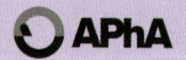

Nutrition *(continued)*

Factors to Consider When Calculating TPN

Factor	Consideration
Macronutrient Complexity	• Consider patient's ability to break down, absorb, & tolerate macronutrients.
Disease Specific	• Consider whether the product is designed for a specific disease state.
Obesity	• ASPEN/SCCM guidelines recommend obese patients (body mass index [BMI] > 30 kg/m^2) should receive 11 to 14 kcal/kg (actual weight) or 22 to 25 kcal/kg (ideal weight); protein requirements should be dosed based upon ideal body weight (IBW).
Allergies	• Lipid emulsion products currently made from soybeans/eggs: contraindicated in patients with severe allergies to soybean/egg.

Note: ASPEN = American Society for Parenteral and Enteral Nutrition; SCCM = Society of Critical Care Medicine.

Refeeding Syndrome

Consideration	Information
Refeeding Syndrome General Information	• Occurs when carbohydrates are introduced to body → insulin to be released & electrolytes to be driven into cells (→ ↓ serum levels)
Risk Factors	• Body mass index (BMI) < 18.5; unintentional weight loss > 10% in 3 months; little/no intake for > 5 days; low electrolyte levels prior to initiation of nutrition therapy
Prevention	• Slow nutrition titration • Close electrolyte monitoring (including K$^+$, Mg^{2+}, & P$^+$) • Patients with refeeding syndrome also experience acute thiamine deficiency due to Krebs cycle; give thiamine to at-risk patients to prevent natural depletion with administration of carbohydrates.
Treatment	• Urgent repletion of electrolytes depending on the severity of lab values (including differences in dosing & formulation)

Reference: Mehanna HM, Moledina J, Travis J. Refeeding syndrome: what it is, and how to prevent and treat it. BMJ 2008;336:1495.

Prepared by Jenna Blunt and Jeanine P. Abrons

Electrolyte & Mineral Requirements— Influences of Needs

Nutrient	Standard Daily Requirement	Factors That ↑ Needs
Calcium*	10 to 15 mEq	High protein intake
Magnesium	8 to 20 mEq	Gastrointestinal (GI) losses; refeeding
Phosphorus*	20 to 40 mmol	High dextrose intake; refeeding
Sodium	1 to 2 mEq/kg*	Diarrhea; vomiting; nasogastric (NG) suction; GI losses
Potassium	1 to 2 mEq/kg*	Diarrhea; vomiting; nasogastric (NG) suction; GI losses; medications; refeeding
Acetate	As needed to maintain acid-base balance	Renal insufficiency; metabolic acidosis; GI losses of bicarbonate
Chloride	As needed to maintain acid-base balance	Metabolic alkalosis; volume depletion

References: ASPEN Guidelines: https://www.nutritioncare.org/Guidelines_and_Clinical_Resources/Clinical_Guidelines/ (Accessed 2021)
*Use caution when calcium and phosphorus are prescribed concurrently as there could be compatibility issues

Clinical Scenario	Formulation Consideration	Example of Formulation Recommendation
High caloric requirement Fluid restriction	Fluid restricted, energy-dense formula	TwoCal® HN
Surgical or trauma patient	Immunomodulating formula	Pivot® 1.5
Persistent diarrhea	Mixed fiber-containing formula	Jevity® 1.5, Osmolite® 1.5
Malabsorption Lack of response to fiber	Small-peptide formula	Pivot® 1.5 CAL, Vital® AF 1.2
Renal impairment	Electrolyte-altered formula	Nepro®
Hyperglycemia	Calorically dense	Glucerna® 1.2
None of the above	Standard formula	Osmolite® 1.2

Card by Jenna Blunt

Chronic Kidney Disease

Chronic Kidney Disease (CKD) Staging

Stage	GFR*	Terminology	Management
G1	≥ 90	Kidney damage with normal/increased GFR	Diagnosis & treatment of comorbid conditions; ↓ progression; cardiovascular risk reduction
G2	60 to 89	Mild reduction in GFR	Estimating progression
G3a	45 to 59	Mild to moderate reduction in GFR	Evaluating & treating complications
G3b	30 to 44	Moderate to severe decrease in GFR*	
G4	15 to 29	Severe reduction in GFR	Preparation for replacement therapy
G5	< 15 (dialysis)	Kidney failure	Replacement therapy by dialysis or transplantation (if uremia present)

*GFR = glomerular filtration rate in mL/min/1.73m^2

Initial card by Jessica Ramich; updated by Loc Nguyen

Kidney Function: Urinary Output

Urinary output (UO) serves a vital role in assessing kidney function. It accounts for the difference between the GFR and the rate of tubular reabsorption. UO provides a greater depiction of the kidneys' acute setting.

Age	Urinary Output Range
Infant	**Normal:** 1.5 to 2 mL/kg/hr **Oliguria:** < 1 mL/kg/hr **Anuria:** No – minimal urine output
Children	**Normal:** 1 to 2 mL/kg/hr **Oliguria:** < 1 mL/kg/hr or < 500 mL/1.73m^2/day in older children **Anuria:** No – minimal urine output
Adults	**Normal:** 0.5 to 1.5 mL/kg/hr **Oliguria:** < 0.3 mL/kg/hr or < 500 mL/day **Anuria:** < 50 mL/day

Nephrotoxic Drugs

General Principles in Use of Nephrotoxic Drugs in CKD:

- Use caution as these agents cause further damage.
- Consider dose reduction or selection of alternative agent.
- Monitor progression of CKD to determine when risk of use of agents outweighs benefits.

Medications with Greater Risk for Nephrotoxicity	
• Aminoglycosides	• Non-steroidal anti-inflammatory drugs
• Amphotericin B	• Polymyxins
• Cisplatin	• Radiographic contrast dye
• Cyclosporine	• Tacrolimus
• Loop diuretics	• Vancomycin

Card content on Nephrotoxic Drugs by Loc Nguyen.

Chronic Kidney Disease *(continued)*

Management of Comorbid Conditions with CKD

Condition	Goal	Cautionary Notes*
Diabetes	**Hemoglobin (Hgb):** $A_{1c} \sim 7\%$	• Recommended use of SGL2 inhibitors • Avoid renally excreted sulfonylureas • Consider dose reduction in insulin when GFR < 30 • Review use of metformin when GFR 30 to 45
Hypertension	**Blood pressure (BP):** < 140/90 mmHg	• Avoid in people with suspected functional renal artery stenosis • If established on therapy, do not routinely discontinue if GFR ↓ < 30 as they remain nephroprotective

Proteinuria	**Protein:** < 3 mg/mmol	• Recommended to use urine albumin-to-creatinine ratio (ACR), or similar available form, for initial testing of proteinuria
		• **Categories:**
		   ◦ A1 (Normal to mildly increased < 3 mg/mmol)
		   ◦ A2 (Moderately increased 3 to 30 mg/mmol)
		   ◦ A3 (Severely increased > 30 mg/mmol)

GFR = glomerular filtration rate in mL/min/1.73m². Recommended to obtain baseline renal function and start at lower doses in the management of comorbidities.

Card by Loc Nguyen

Condition	Goal	Cautionary Notes*
Dyslipidemia	**Low-Density Lipoprotein (LDL):** < 100 mg/dL **Triglycerides (TG):** < 150 mg/dL	• No increase in toxicity for simvastatin dosed at 20 mg/day or simvastatin 20 mg / ezetimibe 10 mg combinations per day when GFR < 30 or on dialysis • The use of fenofibrate increases Serum Creatinine (SCr) by ~0.13 mg/dL.
Anemia	**Hemoglobin (Hgb):** > 11 g/dL	• Frequency of evaluation to be determined by CKD staging • Iron replacement therapy is often effective in anemia. Iron administration to be determined in goals-of-care discussion • ESA** is not recommended in those with active or recent history of malignancy.
Metabolic Bone Disease	**Calcium (Ca^{2+}):** 8.4 to 9.5 mg/dL **Phosphate (PO$_4^{3-}$):** Varies by stage *Stages 3 & 4:* 2.7 to 4.6 mg/dL *Stage 5:* 3.5 to 5.4 mg/dL	• If GFR < 45, recommend measuring serum levels of Ca^{2+}, PO$_4^{3-}$, PTH, and alkaline phosphatase activity at least once • Suggest against the prescription of bisphosphonate in patients with GFR < 30 without a strong clinical rationale

* GFR = glomerular filtration rate in mL/min/1.73m². Recommended to obtain baseline renal function and start at lower doses in the management of comorbidities.
** ESA = Erythropoiesis-Stimulating Agent

Initial card by Jessica Ramich; updated by Loc Nguyen

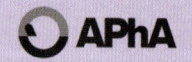

Chronic Kidney Disease *(continued)*

Metabolic Disturbances in CKD

Problem	Intervention	Agents	Dosing
Hyperkalemia	Myocardial stabilization	Calcium gluconate	IV: 1.5 to 3g over 2 to 5 minutes
	Drive K+ intracellularly	Beta-agonist Insulin	Nebulized albuterol 10 to 20 mg over 10 mins Continuous infusion: 1 unit/hour* after IV bolus of dextrose 25 g
	Eliminate K+	Sodium Polystyrene Sulfonate (SPS, kayexalate) Diuretics (Loop)	Oral: 15 g 1 to 4 times daily Rectal: 30 to 50 g every 6 hours IV Furosemide: dose dependent
Hypermagnesemia	Discontinue all sources of magnesium (Milk of Magnesia [MOM], multivitamins, etc.)		
Hyperphosphatemia	Phosphate binders	Aluminum hydroxide, Calcium acetate, Sevelamer	Aluminum hydroxide: Oral: 300 to 600 mg TID with meals Calcium acetate: Oral: 1334 mg with meal, gradual ↑ Sevelamer: Oral: 800 to 1600 mg TID, dependent on level
Hypocalcemia	Supplementation	$CaCO_3$ (use corrected calcium equation)	Oral: 500 mg to 4 g/day in 1 to 3 divided doses
Hyperparathyroidism	Vitamin D analogues Calcium mimetic	Calcitriol Cinacalcet	Oral: 0.25 to 2 mcg/day Oral: 30 to 90 mg 1 to 4 times daily
Metabolic Acidosis	Bicarbonate supplement	Sodium bicarbonate or Sodium citrate/citric acid (Bicitra)	Oral: 650 mg 2 to 3 times daily Oral: 10 to 30 mL QID

Note: Dosing may vary dependent upon institution-specific practice and guidelines. Typical dosing ranges are provided for some agents—consult local practice before making recommendation.
*Infuse to maintain blood glucose of 120 to 180 mg/dL

Card by Loc Nguyen

References
1. Kidney Disease: Improving Global Outcomes (KDIGO) CKD Work Group. "KDIGO 2012 Clinical Practice Guideline for the Evaluation and Management of Chronic Kidney Disease." Kidney inter., Suppl. 2013;3:1–150.
2. CA Johnson, AS Levey, J Coresh, et al. "Clinical practice guidelines for chronic kidney disease in adults: Part I. Definition, disease stages, evaluation, treatment, and risk factors." Am Fam Physician. 2004 Sep 1;70(5):869–76.
3. Monica E. Kleinman, et al. "Part 14: pediatric advanced life support: 2010 American Heart Association guidelines for cardiopulmonary resuscitation and emergency cardiovascular care." Circulation 122.18_suppl_3 (2010):S876–S908.
4. American Academy of Pediatrics Textbook of Pediatric Care. Accessed [October 2021].
5. American Diabetes Association. "Pharmacologic Approaches to Glycemic Treatment: Standards of Medical Care in Diabetes-2020." Diabetes Care 43.Suppl 1 (2020):S98.

Pain Management

World Health Organization Treatment Ladder

Step 1
Mild to Moderate Pain:
Use non-opioid analgesics
(e.g., acetaminophen, nonsteroidal anti-inflammatories)
± adjuvant analgesics

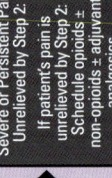

Step 2
Moderate or Persistent Pain Unrelieved by Step 1:
If patient's pain is unrelieved by Step 1: Use low-dose opioid therapy ± non-opioids ± adjuvant analgesics

Step 3
Severe or Persistent Pain Unrelieved by Step 2:
If patient's pain is unrelieved by Step 2: Schedule opioids ± non-opioids ± adjuvant analgesics

Possible Examples of Integrative Therapies
physical therapy, massage, mindfulness, yoga, and others

Term	Definition	Examples
Non-opioids	Pain medications often used in the treatment of mild to moderate pain that do not have opioid properties.	Acetaminophen; ibuprofen; naproxen; salsalate, diflunisal; aspirin
Opioids	A type of medication related to opium with analgesic properties.	Morphine, codeine, oxycodone, hydromorphone, buprenorphine, methadone, fentanyl, oxymorphone, hydrocodone, tramadol, tapentadol
Adjuvant-Neuropathic pain	Drugs primarily indicated for other conditions but found to have benefit in pain management.	Antidepressants (e.g., serotonin norepinephrine uptake inhibitors, tricyclic antidepressants); calcium channel alpha 2-delta ligands (e.g., gabapentin, pregabalin); topical therapy (e.g., lidocaine); sodium channel blockers (e.g., carbamazepine, oxcarbazepine)

Common Adverse Effects of Opioids:
Constipation, nausea/vomiting, sedation, cognitive impairment, pruritus, dry mouth

Other Possible Adverse Effects of Opioids:
Respiratory depression, dependence, anaphylaxis, seizures, urinary retention, delirium, hyperalgesia opioid-induced androgen deficiency, osteoporosis, apnea, immunosuppression

Pain Assessment Tools:
- 0 to 10 numeric rating scale (NRS)
- Wong-Baker FACES® Pain Rating Scale: http://wongbakerfaces.org/ (Accessed 2019)
- Visual analog scale (VAS)
- COMFORT scale
- CRIES scale (crying, oxygenation, vital signs, facial expression, & sleeplessness) (Pediatric)
- MOBID-2 (dementia)
- FLACC (face, legs, activity, cry, & consolability) score
- Brief pain inventory (BPI)

Resources
- Schneider C, Yale SH, Larson M. Principles of Pain Management. *Clin Med Res*. 2003. 1(4): 337–340.
- National Institutes of Health (NIH): Pain Consortium: https://painconsortium.nih.gov/ (Accessed 2021)
- American Academy of Pain Medicine: https://painmed.org/clinician-resource-for-pain-medicine (Accessed 2020)
- JAMA Patient Page: Acute Pain Treatment. *JAMA*. 2008. 299(1):128.
- Agency Medical Directors Group. Interagency Guideline on Opioid Dosing for Chronic Non-Cancer Pain (CNCP). 2010.
- Equianalgesic Dosing of Opioids for Pain Management. Pharmacist's Letter. August 2012.
- Gippsland Region Palliative Care Consortium Clinical Practice Group. Opioid Conversion Guidelines. February 2011.
- https://www.cdc.gov/drugoverdose/pdf/calculating_total_daily_dose-a.pdf (Accessed 2021)

Dosages at or above 50 morphine milligram equivalents (MME)/day ↑ risks for respiratory depression by at least 2 times

Updated by Jeanine Abrons and Kashelle Lockman

Co-Prescribing Naloxone for Outpatient Settings

Use of Naloxone:

- Naloxone ↓ overdose deaths & ↑ engagement in substance use disorder (SUD) treatment among persons with SUD. It also decreases emergency department visits for respiratory depression in patients taking chronic opioids for pain. Overall, there should be a low threshold for recommending naloxone for emergency use.
- In 2020, the FDA required labeling changes to opioids & medications for opioid use disorder (OUD) to recommend that naloxone discussion, education, and risk-factor-driven co-prescribing be a routine part of opioid & MOUD prescribing.

Risk Factors for Severe Respiratory Depression from Opioids:

Patients can experience severe respiratory depression from opioids for a variety of reasons, including frail physiology; The following risk factors for opioid-induced respiratory depression have been noted in studies:[1-5]

• Male gender[2] • Age > 65 years old[1] or age 45 to 54 years old[2] • History of SUD including tobacco or alcohol[1] • Poverty[2] • Renal dysfunction[1] • Multiple prescribers[1] • Alcohol[1] • Recently incarcerated or in treatment facility with history of opioid use disorder[1] • History of opioid overdose[1] • Neuropsychiatric illness[1] • Hepatic dysfunction[1]	• Benzodiazepines[4] • Alcohol[1] • Non-benzodiazepine (BZD) sedative hypnotics[2] • Gabapentin ≥ 900 mg total daily dose (TDD)[3] • Pregabalin[5] • Skeletal muscle relaxants[2] • Antidepressants[2] • Oral morphine equivalents (OME) ≥ 50 mg[1] • Opioid conversions[1] • Extended release (ER) opioids[2] • Skeletal muscle relaxants[2] • Non-benzodiazepine (BZD) sedative hypnotics[2] • Gabapentin ≥ 900 mg total daily dose (TDD)[3] • Opioid treatment > 31 days[2]

Tools & Calculators for Estimating Risk of Opioid-Induced Respiratory Depression or Overdose:

Several tools and calculators have been developed to integrate patient- and medication-related risk factors to evaluate a patient's relative risk of overdose and/or serious opioid-induced respiratory depression. Published, peer-reviewed tools include:

- Risk Index for Serious Opioid-Induced Respiratory Depression (RIOSORD) for Civilians[6] & Veterans[7]
- Stratification Tool for Opioid Risk Mitigation (STORM) for Veterans[8]
- Kaiser Model[9]

In addition, Appriss Health includes a proprietary Overdose Risk Score (ORS) in its PMP, which is used in 52 US states and territories.[10,11] The score provided by this tool does not factor in clinical indicators or drug/formulation-specific variables.

Other Practical Reasons to Consider Naloxone in an Outpatient Setting:

- When high-risk age groups (e.g., teenagers) live in or visit the patient's home or if the patient lives in a remote location.
- The Centers for Disease Control and Prevention (CDC) & the American Medical Association (AMA) recommend considering prescribing naloxone for the following conditions:

CDC	AMA
• History of substance use disorder (SUD) • History of overdose • Concomitant benzodiazepine use • Risk of returning to a high dose when no longer opioid tolerant • ≥ 50 mg oral morphine equivalence daily dose (MEDD)	• High-dose opioids • History of SUD • Mental health condition • Respiratory disease; sleep apnea • Concomitant benzodiazepine use • Person in a position to assist

Modifying Patient Risk Factors for Severe Respiratory Depression:

- If your patient has risk factors:
  - Remove that risk factor if possible by optimizing drug therapy through drug selection or careful deprescribing.
  - If a risk factor isn't modifiable, consider recommending naloxone based on any risk factors for severe respiratory depression, using your clinical judgment.

Similarities and Differences Between Naloxone Formulations

Factors consistent between all products:
- Two refills available on all products
- Repeat administration after two to three minutes if no/minimal response
- FDA approved

Product/NDC	Supplied as	Assembly	Dose Titration	Storage Temp	Initial Administration*	Website
Injectable/intranasal generic NDC:76329-3369-01 2 mg/2 mL	• Two 2 mL luer-lock needleless syringes plus two mucosal atomizers	Y	Y	59 to 86°F	Spray 1 mL (1/2 of syringe) in one nostril. Repeat in other nostril if no/minimal response.	Amphastar.com OR Teleflex.com
Narcan** 4 mg/0.1 mL [NDC: 69547-353-02]	• 4 mg/0.1 mL: Two-pack	N	N	59 to 77°F*	Spray 0.1 mL into one nostril. Repeat in other nostril if no/minimal response.	Narcannalspray.com
Injectable generic 0.4 mg/mL or 4 mg/10 mL NDC: Varied—Pfizer, Mylan, & West-Ward	• Two single-use 1 mL vials; two 3 mL syringes with 23- to 25-gauge, 1 to 1.5 in. IM needles • One 10 mL multidose vial, two 3 mL syringes with 23- to 25-gauge 1 to 1.5 in. IM needles	Y	Y	68 to 77°F	Inject 1 mL in shoulder or thigh.	Pfizerinjectables.com OR Mylan.com OR West-ward.com

* = excursions from 41°F to 104°F
** = generics approved by FDA in 2019 with unknown date of availability in market
Adapted from Prescribe to Prevent. "Naloxone Product Comparison Table." PrescribeToPrevent.org (Accessed December 2021)

Created by Kashelle Lockman

Recommending Naloxone to a Patient

Studies show patients appreciate the offer of naloxone if it is presented as a universal precaution, similar to fire extinguishers and safety belts. (Hope for the best; plan for the rest.) The following scripts may be helpful to recommend naloxone to a patient. If the patient agrees, comprehensive counseling on naloxone use should be included at the time of dispensing.

If patient is taking prescribed chronic opioid therapy:

- Opioids are strong pain medicines that can slow or stop breathing.
- Taking opioids as your physician or healthcare professional tells you lowers the chance this will happen, but sometimes our bodies respond to medicines in unexpected ways.
- This might happen if you become sick, start other medicines that also slow breathing, or take too much opioids. This can happen at any point in treatment, whether you are new to opioids or have been taking them for months to years.
- Naloxone is a medicine that can temporarily restart your breathing and wake you up if your body ever responds to opioids in this way.
- Having naloxone in your home is like having a fire extinguisher. It is only for rare emergencies.
- If opioids ever make you stop breathing, you won't be able to give naloxone to yourself.
- Share the instructions on using it with a friend or loved one who would be able to help you if this emergency ever happens.

If patient has an active substance use disorder (SUD) or history of one, be sure to reassure them that you want them to have naloxone because you care.

You may also want to add:

- I talk to all of my patients who take opioids for medical conditions about naloxone.
- If you ever need to use this, please let us know so we can refill it for you.
- If the cost of naloxone is a financial burden for you, I can look for a coupon or refer you to a program that may provide free naloxone.
- Naloxone will not harm a person if the patient is not experiencing an overdose (e.g., collapsed from cardiac arrest, not an OD).

Naloxone should not be used as a condition of filling an opioid prescription. There are many reasons a patient may not accept an offer of naloxone, including but not limited to:

- Stigma
- Cost
- Lack of caregiver to administer it.

Kashelle Lockman

Recommending Naloxone to a Patient *(continued)*

- **I: Identify** the need for naloxone. A person who needs naloxone may have very slow/no breathing, no response to shouting or firmly rubbing your fist over their breastbone, cold, &/or blue/purplish hands and feet, and pinpoint pupils.
- **C: Call** 911. Naloxone will wear off in as little as 30 minutes.
- **A: Administer** naloxone (see naloxone formulation table for product-specific instructions) and provide **airway breathing** after ensuring nothing is in the person's mouth.
- **R: Redose** naloxone in 2 to 3 minutes if the person still isn't awake. **Restart** airway breathing.
- **E: Ensure** the person's safety until emergency responders arrive. Lay them on their side in case they vomit. Don't let them take more opioids. Reassure them help is on the way. They may have a fast heart rate, runny nose, sneezing, shivering, sweating, diarrhea, pain, and irritability.

References Related to Naloxone & Opioid-Induced Respiratory Depression or Overdose:

1. Dowell D, Haegerich TM, Chou R. CDC Guideline for Prescribing Opioids for Chronic Pain—United States, 2016. JAMA. 2016;315(15):1624. doi:10.1001/jama.2016.1464
2. Garg RK, Fulton-Kehoe D, Franklin GM. Patterns of Opioid Use and Risk of Opioid Overdose Death Among Medicaid Patients. Med Care. 2017;55(7):661–668. doi:10.1097/MLR.0000000000000738
3. Gomes T, Juurlink DN, Antoniou T, Mamdani MM, Paterson JM, van den Brink W. Gabapentin, opioids, and the risk of opioid-related death: A population-based nested Case–control study. Tsai AC, ed. PLOS Med. 2017;14(10):e1002396. doi:10.1371/journal.pmed.1002396
4. Park TW, Saitz R, Ganoczy D, Ilgen MA, Bohnert ASB. Benzodiazepine prescribing patterns and deaths from drug overdose among US veterans receiving opioid analgesics: Case-cohort study. Bmj. 2015;350(jun10 9):h2698–h2698. doi:10.1136/bmj.h2698
5. Gomes T, Greaves S, van den Brink W, et al. Pregabalin and the Risk for Opioid-Related Death: A Nested Case-Control Study. Ann Intern Med. 2018;169(10):732–734. doi:10.7326/M14
6. Zedler BK, Saunders WB, Joyce AR, Vick CC, Murrelle EL. Validation of a Screening Risk Index for Serious Prescription Opioid-Induced Respiratory Depression or Overdose in a US Commercial Health Plan Claims Database. Pain Med. March 2017. doi:10.1093/pm/pnx009
7. Zedler B, Xie L, Wang L, et al. Development of a Risk Index for Serious Prescription Opioid-Induced Respiratory Depression or Overdose in Veterans' Health Administration Patients. Pain Med. 2015;16(8):1566–579. doi:10.1111/pme.12777
8. Oliva EM, Christopher MLD, Wells D, et al. Opioid overdose education and naloxone distribution: Development of the Veterans Health Administration's national program Veterans Health Administration Opioid Overdose Education and Naloxone Distribution National Support and Development Workgroup. J Am Pharm Assoc. 2017;57:S168–S179.e4. doi:10.1016/j.japh.2017.01.022
9. Glanz JM, Narwaney KJ, Mueller SR, et al. Prediction Model for Two-Year Risk of Opioid Overdose Among Patients Prescribed Chronic Opioid Therapy. J Gen Intern Med. 2018;33(10):1646–1653. doi:10.1007/s11606-017-4288-3
10. Huizenga J, Breneman B, VR P, A R, DB S. NARxCHECK Score as a Predictor of Unintentional Overdose Death.; 2016.
11. Appriss Health: Iowa PMP Aware User Support Manual. http://pharmacy.iowa.gov/sites/default/files/documents/2018/04/ia_pmp_awarexe_requestor_user_manual.pdf (Accessed 2021)

Kashelle Lockman

Veterinary Medicine Information

Veterinary Consideration	Description
Counseling	**Insulin Administration Technique** • Inject at a 45° angle under skin around neck of a dog or cat (e.g., where a mom cat carries her kittens). • Keep needle parallel to skin & inject under loose skin between neck & back. • Subcutaneous is preferred; intramuscular (IM) administration is an option (administer IM in thigh) but not preferred due to nerve damage risk. ○ Further details: https://www.petcoach.co/ (Accessed 2020) **SIG Abbreviations** • Vary for humans & animals (e.g., once daily: humans = QD; animals = SID)
Dosing Considerations	• Pain medications/antibiotics dosed higher (different from humans). • Dosing is usually weight based.
Toxicity	• Ingestion (accidental or overdose) of some OTC products may be toxic to pets. • Xylitol: A common ingredient in chocolate, sugar free gum, and liquid medication formulations is lethal to dogs **Most common OTC medications that are potentially toxic to pets:** • Acetaminophen • Naproxen • Ibuprofen *Note: May be dose dependent* **Most common prescription medications that are potentially toxic to pets:** • ACE Inhibitors • Duloxetine • Alprazolam • Tramadol • Amphetamine salts • Venlafaxine • Beta blockers • Zolpidem • Clonazepam
Compounding	• FDA Regulations & Compliance Policy Guide 608.400 "Compounding of Drugs for Use in Animals." • Veterinary medicines may be compounded when no approved animal or human drug is available. • ***Compounding related resource:*** American Veterinary Medical Association—Compounding: https://www.avma.org/KB/Policies/Pages/Compounding.aspx

Drug, Dosing, & Pharmacology Resources
- Plumb's Veterinary Drug Handbook (primary resource for veterinary care)
- National Animal Poison Control Center: www.aspca.org/pet-care/poison-control
- American Veterinary Medical Association—Compounding: https://www.avma.org/KB/Policies/Pages/Compounding.aspx and https://www.avma.org/resources-tools/avma-policies/guidelines-veterinary-prescription-drugs
- FDA Guidelines and Regulations for Veterinary Prescriptions: https://www.fda.gov/animal-veterinary/guidance-regulations
- DVM 360: https://www.dvm360.com/view/guidelines-veterinary-clinical-practice - links to numerous veterinary guidelines
- "Green Book" online: https://animaldrugsatfda.fda.gov/adafda/views/#/search - Approved animal products in a searchable database; can search by different criteria (e.g., indications, approved species, ingredients, etc.)
- Drugs.com: https://www.drugs.com/vet/ - Has a database of veterinary products from many different manufacturers
- Compendium of Veterinary Products (CVP): https://vayerall.cvpservice.com/ - Allows you to search for information about veterinary pharmaceuticals, other products, biologicals, and withdrawal time charts
- The Merck Veterinary Manual: https://merckvetmanual.com/ - Divided by system, then by disease; includes reference guide tables for specific tests and measures.
- USP Veterinary Clinical Drug Information Monographs: Monographs developed by the USP and the Veterinary Drug Expert Committee.
- https://dailymed.nlm.nih.gov/dailymed/

Veterinary Disease States
- www.Petplace.com

Legal & Regulatory Resources
- Food & Drug Association (FDA)/Center for Veterinary Medicine (CVM): http://www.fda.gov/AnimalVeterinary

Poison Control
- Animal Poison Control Center: (855) 764-7661
- ASPCA Animal Poison Control Center Phone Number: (888) 426-4435

Revised by Marissa Rupalo

Transplant Medications

Maintenance Agents

- All dosing & target trough levels should be based on the organ transplanted, the time since transplantation, and the patient's risk of rejection and infection

Drug	Dosing	Drug Level Monitoring	Adverse Effects#	Common Drug Interactions/Notes
Calcineurin Inhibitors				
Tacrolimus* (Prograf®, Astagraf XL®, Envarsus XR®)	**Starting doses:** • **IR:** 0.05 to 0.15 mg/kg/day PO divided every 12 hours 　○ Can be given SL: starting dose is 1/2 the PO dose • **IV:** 0.01 to 0.05 mg/kg/day continuous infusion based on type of transplant* • **XL:** 0.1 to 0.2 mg/kg PO daily • **XR:** 0.14 mg/kg PO daily 　○ IR:XR dose conversion ratio is 1 mg : 0.7 mg XR and 1:0.85 for African American patients 　○ IV tacrolimus is not typically used first but rather converted to it if a patient is not able to take orally & are not therapeutic 　○ IV to PO conversion = 1/3 to 1/4 total daily oral adult dose (conversion may differ between centers)	**Trough levels:** 4 to 15 ng/ml	**Class effects:** • Nephrotoxicity • Hypertension • Hyperlipidemia • Hyperglycemia • Hyperkalemia **Unique to this drug within the class:** • QTc prolongation • Alopecia • Posterior reversible encephalopathy syndrome (PRES) • Tremor • Headache	• 3A4 inducers or inhibitors • Live vaccines*** • Nephrotoxic agents (e.g., aminoglycosides, vancomycin)
Cyclosporine** (Sandimmune®) Cyclosporine modified (Gengraf®, Neoral®)	**Starting doses:** • **PO:** 10 to 15 mg/kg/day PO divided every 12 hours • **IV (Sandimmune):** 5 to 6 mg/kg/day or 1/3 of the total oral dose	**Trough levels:** 100 to 300ng/ml	**Class effects:** • See above **Unique to this drug within the class:** • Progressive multifocal leukoencephalopathy (PML) • Hepatotoxicity • Gingival hyperplasia • Hirsutism acne • Acne	• 3A4 inducers or inhibitors • Live vaccines • Nephrotoxic agents

*Notes: # the table is a list of adverse effects not inclusive of all possible adverse effects; * Tacrolimus IR, XL & XR products are not interchangeable; ** not interchangeable with cyclosporine modified; *** avoidance of live vaccines is a general rule in an immunosuppressed state, not an interaction with a specific medication. IR = immediate release; XL and XR = extended release formulations; IV = intravenous; PO = by mouth; BID = twice daily.*

Prepared by Erica Maceira and Vassilia Sideras

Transplant Medications (continued)

Drug	Dosing	Drug Level Monitoring	Adverse Effects*	Common Drug Interactions/Notes
Antiproliferative/Antimetabolite Agents				
Mycophenolate (Cellcept®, Myfortic®)*	**Starting doses:** • Mycophenolate mofetil: 1 to 1.5 g IV/PO BID • Mycophenolic acid: 360 mg to 720 mg PO BID	Use of monitoring mycophenolic acid plasma levels or AUC is not well defined & not routinely advised	**Class effects:** • Anemia • Thrombocytopenia • Neutropenia • PML **Unique to this drug within the class:** • Teratogenic, ↑ risk of 1st trimester pregnancy loss • Edema • Pleural effusion • Diarrhea • Hypertension • Hyperglycemia	• Magnesium • Aluminum • Cholestyramine • Proton pump inhibitors • Rifampin • Rifabutin • Live vaccines **Bullet–Associated REMS–requires two forms of birth control in women of child bearing potential**
Azathioprine (Imuran®)	**Starting doses:** • 2 to 5 mg/kg/PO initially then 1 to 3 mg/kg PO daily • 50 to 150 mg daily	Not applicable (N/A)	**Unique to this drug within the class:** • Leukopenia • Thrombocytopenia • Anemia • Nausea • Vomiting • Hepatotoxicity (< 1%) • Veno-occlusive liver disease • PML	• Allopurinol, febuxostat – contraindicated • Live vaccines

Notes: *Products are not interchangeable. AUC = area under the curve; IV = intravenous; PO = by mouth; BID = twice daily; not inclusive of all side effects; REMS = Risk Evaluation and Mitigation Strategies

Transplant Medications *(continued)*

Drug	Dosing	Drug Level Monitoring	Adverse Effects[a]	Common Drug Interactions/Notes
mTOR Inhibitors				
Sirolimus (Rapamune®)	**Starting doses:** • 3 mg/m^2 (Max: 15 mg) PO Post operative day one (POD1) **Maintenance:** • 1 mg/m^2 (Max: 5 mg) PO daily	**Trough levels:** • 4 to 15 ng/mL	**Class effects:** • Anemia • Thrombocytopenia • Interstitial lung disease • Stomatitis • Acne • Hyperlipidemia • Hypertriglyceridemia • Peripheral edema • Lymphocele • Impaired wound healing • Pericardial effusions • Angioedema **Unique to this drug within the class:** • Avoid use with liver transplant: ↑ risk of hepatic artery thrombosis, graft loss, & ↑ mortality when used with cyclosporine or tacrolimus	• Strong CYP3A4 &/or P-glycoprotein inhibitors or inducers • Live vaccines
Everolimus (Zortress®)	**Starting doses:** • 0.75 to 1 mg PO BID	**Trough levels:** • 3 to 8 ng/mL	**Class effects:** • See above **Unique to this drug within the class:** • Hypertension • Hypophosphatemia	• Strong CYP3A4 &/or P-glycoprotein inhibitors or inducers • Live vaccines

Notes: PO = by mouth; BID = twice daily; not inclusive of all side effects

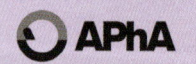

Transplant Medications *(continued)*

Drug	Dosing	Drug Level Monitoring	Adverse Effects#	Common Drug Interactions/Notes
Steroids				
Prednisone	**Starting doses:** • 5 to 20 mg PO daily	N/A	**Class effects:** • Hypertension • Fluid retention • Impaired glucose tolerance • ↑ Appetite • Weight gain • Osteoporosis • Mood changes • GI perforation • Hypokalemia • Hypocalcemia	• Aspirin • Quinolones: ↑ risk of tendon rupture • Hormonal contraceptives: Potential ↓ efficacy • NSAIDs: ↑ risk of GI ulcers/bleeding • Live vaccines
Co-stimulation Blocker				
Belatacept (Nulojix®) *Patients must be EBV seropositive to receive*	**Starting doses:** • Day 1 (day of transplant) & 5; end of weeks 2, 4, 8, & 12: 10 mg/kg IV • 5 mg/kg at end of week 16 then every 4 weeks **Conversion:** • 5 mg/kg IV ~ every 2 weeks until day 57, then every 4 weeks	N/A	**Unique to this drug within the class:** • Hypertension • Dyslipidemia • Peripheral edema • Posttransplant lymphoproliferative disorder (particularly CNS) in patients who are EBV seronegative	• Live vaccines

Notes: CNS = central nervous system; EBV = Epstein-Barr virus; GI = gastrointestinal; IV = intravenous; NSAIDs = non-steroidal anti-inflammatory drugs; PO = by mouth; # not inclusive of all side effects

Transplant Medications *(continued)*

Induction Agents

Drug	Dosing	Adverse Effects[a]
Antithymocyte globulin, rabbit (Thymoglobulin®)	• **IV:** 1.5 mg/kg IV daily for 3 to 7 days • Pre-medicate with acetaminophen &/or antihistamine (or corticosteroid if not already on) about 30 to 60 minutes prior to infusion • Doses may be adjusted or held (decrease 50% if WBC 2 to 3 and/or platelets 50 to 70; hold if WBC < 2 and/or platelets < 50) based on patient response, white blood count (WBC) ↓ or platelet ↓	**Unique to this drug within the class:** • Infusion reactions (chest pain, dyspnea, chills, anaphylaxis, cytokine release syndrome) • Tachycardia • Hypertension • Leukopenia, anemia, and thrombocytopenia • Reactivation of infections (T-cell depletion)
Alemtuzumab (Campath®) (restricted access)	• **IV:** 30 mg IV once at the time of transplant	**Unique to this drug within the class:** • Infusion reaction (anaphylaxis, angioedema, bronchospasm, hypotension, chest pain, bradycardia, tachycardia, transient neurologic symptoms, hypertension, headache, pyrexia) • Hypersensitivity reaction • Acute cholecystitis • Lymphoproliferative disorder
Basiliximab (Simulect®)	• **IV:** 20 mg IV on day of transplant then 20 mg IV on day 4 • Second dose is withheld if patient had severe hypersensitivity reaction to the initial dose	**Unique to this drug within the class:** • Severe acute hypersensitivity reactions (e.g., anaphylaxis, hypotension, tachycardia, dyspnea, wheezing, pulmonary edema, urticaria, pruritus) • Hypertension • Peripheral edema

Notes: IV = intravenous; not inclusive of all side effects.

Prepared by Erica Maceira and Vassilia Sidera

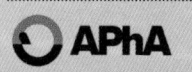

Free Quality Online Resources

Resource	Features or Benefit	Limitations in Use
U.S. Food and Drug Administration (FDA) http://www.fda.gov/	• Animal Drugs@FDA (Green Book) • Therapeutic Equivalence Evaluations (Orange Book) • Drugs@FDA • FDA Drug Shortages • National Drug Code Directory • Database of Licensed Biological Products (Purple Book)	The large amount of information may make navigation difficult.
U.S. National Library of Medicine (NLM) https://www.nlm.nih.gov/	• Drug Information Portal • MEDLINE/PubMed/MedlinePlus • ClinicalTrials.gov • DailyMed • Populations & genetics information • Environmental health & toxicology	The connection or overlap of information between libraries; cross-referencing is improving.
Drugs.com https://www.drugs.com	• ~24,000 monographs from Wolters Kluwer Health, American Society of Health-System Pharmacists, Cerner Multum, & Micromedex from IBM Watson Micromedex	This website may appear cluttered. Commercial advertising is accepted.
Medscape: Drugs & Diseases http://reference.medscape.com	• ~ 7,100 monographs based on FDA approvals • ~ 6,000 peer-reviewed EBP disease & conditions articles	Information is abbreviated & may not be comprehensive.
Merck Manuals http://www.merckmanuals.com/	• Drug monographs from Wolters Kluwer UpToDate, Inc. • Consumer/Professional Version • Veterinary Edition	Publication reflects medical practice & information in the United States. It does not include international perspectives.
Centers for Disease Control and Prevention (CDC) http://www.cdc.gov/	• Morbidity & Mortality Weekly Report • 2020 Childhood & Adult Immunization Schedules • 2020 Yellow Book (Health Information for International Travel) • Free travel apps: TravWell; Can I Eat This?	Lots of information but easy navigation.
Drug Enforcement Administration (DEA) https://www.dea.gov	• 2020 Drugs of Abuse	Focused on enforcement of controlled substances laws & U.S. regulations; not global.
World Health Organization (WHO) http://www.who.int/en/	• International Pharmacopoeia • World Health Statistics • International Travel & Health • International Classification of Diseases-11	The website's expansive coverage makes navigation difficult.
Institute for Safe Medication Practices (ISMP) http://www.ismp.org	• ISMP Guidelines • Medication Error Reporting • Medication safety tools and resources	The organization provides independent oversight. It relies on donations & grants. Subscriptions are fee based.
Agency for Healthcare Research and Quality (AHRQ) http://www.ahrq.gov/	• Pharmacy Health Literacy Center	Lots of information but easy to navigate.

Note: All sites accessed 2021.
Prepared by Vern Duba & Jeanine P. Ahrons

National Clinical Guidelines

Cardiovascular Section Guidelines

Guideline (Publication Date)	Recognized Source of Guideline
Anticoagulation Therapy/ Venous Thromboembolism	American Society of Hematology
Blood Cholesterol (2018)	American College of Cardiology & American Heart Association (ACC/AHA)
Heart Failure (2017 & 2019; 2021) Acute (2014); Chronic (2018)	American College of Cardiology, American Heart Association, & Heart Failure Society of America (ACC/AHA/HFSA); 2021 = European Society of Cardiology National Institute for Health & Care Excellence (NICE)
Hypertension (2017)	American College of Cardiology & American Heart Association (ACC/AHA)
Cardiovascular Disease Prevention Clinical Practice Guidelines	European Society of Cardiology (ESC) published in the European Heart Journal
Myocardial Infarction (MI) (2013, 2014, 2017) Acute Coronary Syndrome Without Persistent ST-segment Elevation (2020)	American College of Cardiology & American Heart Association (ACC/AHA); European Society of Cardiology (ESC) Chest Pain Clinical Practice Guidelines were updated by the Journal of the American College of Cardiology December 2021.
Overweight & Obesity (2013)	American College of Cardiology, American Heart Association, The Obesity Society (ACC/AHA/TOS)
Stroke Prevention (2021) Guidelines also exist for prevention	American Heart Association & American Stroke Association (AHA/ASA)

Note: Individual areas updated separately

Endocrine Section Guidelines

Guideline (Publication Date)	Recognized Source of Guideline
Diabetes (yearly updates)	American Diabetes Association (ADA)
Endocrine (multiple years)	American Association of Clinical Endocrinologists & American College of Endocrinology (AACE/ACE)

Respiratory Section Guidelines

Guideline (Publication Date)	Recognized Source of Guideline
Asthma (GINA 2021; EPR 3 = 2017)	Global Initiative for Asthma (GINA): National Asthma Education & Prevention Program (NAEPP) Expert Panel Report (EPR) 3
Chronic Obstructive Pulmonary Disease (2021)	Global Initiative for Chronic Obstructive Lung Disease (GOLD)

National Clinical Guidelines *(continued)*

Infectious Diseases Section Guidelines

Guideline (Publication Date)	Where to Access
Community-Acquired Pneumonia (CAP) (2019)	Infectious Diseases Society of America
Hospital-Acquired Pneumonia (HAP) & Ventilator-Associated Pneumonia (VAP) (2016)	Infectious Diseases Society of America
Clostridium Difficile (2018)	Infectious Diseases Society of America
Other (multiple years)	Infectious Diseases Society of America

Special Populations Section Guidelines

Guideline (Publication Date)	Where to Access
Beers Criteria (2019)	American Geriatrics Society
Pharmacological Management of Persistent Pain in Older Persons (2009)	American Geriatrics Society
Prevention of Falls in Older Persons (2010)	American Geriatrics Society
Management of Blood Pressure in Chronic Kidney Disease (KDIGO) (2021)	Kidney International

Miscellaneous Section Guidelines

Guideline (Publication Date)	Where to Access
Mental Health	
Alzheimer's Disease (2011)	https://www.alz.org/health-care-professionals/clinical-guidelines-dementia-care.asp

Prepared by Jeanine P. Abrons

Clinically Significant Drug Interactions

Category/ Classification	Electronic Resource
Cytochrome P450 Drug Interactions	Indiana University Division of Clinical Pharmacology P450 Drug Interaction Table *(https://drug-interactions.medicine.iu.edu/)*
QTc-Prolonging Medications	Arizona Center for Education and Research on Therapeutics *(https://www.crediblemeds.org/index.php/login/dlcheck)* Free registration now required
Grapefruit Interactions with Medications	University of Washington *(https://labs.wsu.edu/paine/research/)* National Center for Complementary and Alternative Medicine *(https://nccih.nih.gov/health/providers/digest/herb-drug)* FDA *(http://www.fda.gov/ForConsumers/consumerupdates/ucm292276.htm)* Medscape Drug Interaction Checker *(https://reference.medscape.com/drug-interactionchecker)*
Oral Contraception Interactions/ Pregnancy	Reprotox *(https://www.reprotox.org)* Additional resources listed in "Special Populations" section; Note: paid resource
Herbal Information	National Center for Complementary & Integrative Health *(https://www.nccih.nih.gov/health/herbsataglance)*
Dietary Supplements	National Center for Complementary & Integrative Health *(https://www.nccih.nih.gov/health/using-dietary-supplements-wisely)*

All websites accessed November 2021.
Prepared by Jeanine P. Abrons

Medications with Adverse Withdrawal Effects from Abrupt Discontinuation

Medication Category	Medication Examples	Presentation with Abrupt Stop	Symptoms	Risk Factors/Management	Evidence	Potential to be Life Threatening
Alpha Agonist	Clonidine (Catapres®)	Rebound hypertension; tachycardia; agitation; headache; nervousness; stroke (rarely): encephalopathy (rarely)	Mild to Severe	• **Risk factor** - Use > 1 month, cardiovascular disease. β-blocker use, daily dose > 1.2 mg • **Management** - Taper over 6 to 10 days by ↓ dose by one-third to one-half every 2 to 3 days	Excellent	YES
Anticonvulsant	Gabapentin (Neurontin®) Pregabalin (Lyrica®) Phenytoin (Dilantin®) Topiramate (Topamax®)	Seizures (and increasing frequency of); anxiety, insomnia; nausea; pain; sweating	Mild to Severe	• **Management** - Taper over at least 2 to 4 weeks Topiramate: ↓ by 50-100mg for seizures and ↓ by 25-50mg for migraine prophylaxis over 2-8 weeks	Good	YES
Antidepressant	Desvenlafaxine (Pristiq®) Duloxetine (Cymbalta®) Paroxetine (Paxil®) Sertraline (Zoloft®) Venlafaxine (Effexor®)	Flulike symptoms; insomnia; nausea; imbalance; sensory disturbances; hyper-arousal (FINISH); lethargy; dizziness; anxiety; irritability; vivid dreams; headache; abdominal pain; diarrhea	Mild to Moderate	• **Risk factors** - > 6 weeks use or short T½ - Prior history of antidepressant withdrawal symptoms; ↑ doses of drug • **Management** - ↓ dose over weeks to months - Sub longer acting agent & ↓ every 2 to 3 weeks. - ↓ based on indication	Good	NO
Anti-Parkinson	Amantadine (Symmetrel®) Carbidopa/Levodopa (Sinemet®) Rasagiline (Azilect®)	Hyperpyrexia; confusion; muscle rigidity; tachycardia; tachypnea	Severe	• **Management** - Taper over ~ 4 weeks	Good	YES
Antipsychotic	Clozapine (Clozaril®) Haloperidol (Haldol®) Olanzapine (Zyprexa®) Quetiapine (Seroquel®) Risperidone (Risperdal®)	Sweating; salivation; flu symptoms; paresthesia; bronchoconstriction; urination; gastrointestinal; anorexia; vertigo; insomnia, agitation/ anxiety; restlessness; movement disorders, psychosis	Mild to Severe	• **Management** - No > 50% ↓ every 2 weeks - May stop more abruptly in hospital - If switching agent, may cross-taper: ↓ dose of old agent while titrating up new agent at ~ same rate (e.g., over 2 to 3 weeks)	Excellent	NO

Updated by Crystal McElhose; previous updates by Angela Wojtczak, Joanna Rusch, Elisha Andreas, and Jeanine P. Abrons.

Medications with Adverse Withdrawal Effects from Abrupt Discontinuation *(continued)*

Medication Category	Medication Examples	Presentation with Abrupt Stop	Symptoms	Risk Factors/Management	Evidence	Potential to be Life Threatening
Benzodiazepine and "Z drugs"	Alprazolam (Xanax®) Clonazepam (Klonopin®) Eszopiclone (Lunesta®) Lorazepam (Ativan®) Triazolam (Halcion) Zolpidem (Ambien)	Sweating; tremor; agitation; nausea; tachycardia; insomnia; anxiety; vomiting; hallucinations; seizures	Mild to Severe	• **Risk factors** · High-dose, long-term use · Use of short-acting agent • **Management** · Taper or sub long-acting agent over 2 to 3 months	Excellent	YES
Beta Blocker	Atenolol (Tenormin®) Bisoprolol (Zebeta®) Metoprolol (multiple) Propranolol (Inderal®)	Hypertension; angina; myocardial infarction; ventricular arrhythmia	Mild to Severe	• **Management** · ↓ dosage over 1 to 2 weeks & up to 3 weeks with history of myocardial infarction	Good	YES
Butalbital Combination Products	Fiorinal Fioricet	Headache exacerbation; delirium; tremors; seizures	Mild to Severe	• **Risk factor** · Constant, long-term use of ≥ 7 doses daily • **Management** · Taper over 4 to 6 weeks. With ≥ 12 doses daily, consider referral.	Fair	YES
Carbamate	Carisoprodol (Soma®)	Body aches; sweats; palpitations; anxiety; restlessness; insomnia	Mild to Moderate	• **Management** · Long taper: renal or liver impairment, age > 65, TDD > 1400 mg, taper over 9 days* (specific taper schedule available) · Short taper: taper over 4 days*	Fair	NO
Corticosteroid	Hydrocortisone (Cortef®) Methylprednis (Solu-Medrol®) Prednisone (Deltasone®)	Adrenal insufficiency—nausea; vomiting; fatigue; weakness, ↓ appetite; ↓ weight; hypoglycemia; ↓ mood; adrenal crisis	Mild to Severe	• **Risk factor** · Prednisone > 7.5 mg daily for ≥ 3 weeks • **Management** · Based on institution; taper over 2 months for pituitary-adrenal response recovery	Excellent	YES

Updated by Crystal McElhose; previous updates by Angela Wojtczak, Joanna Rusch, Elisha Andreas, and Jeanine P. Abrons.

Medications with Adverse Withdrawal Effects from Abrupt Discontinuation *(continued)*

Medication Category	Medication Examples	Presentation with Abrupt Stop	Symptoms	Risk Factors/Management	Evidence	Potential to be Life Threatening
Nitrate	Isosorbide mononitrate & dinitrate (Imdur®, Isordil®)	Rebound angina	Mild to Severe	**Management** • Consider taper over 1 to 2 weeks, use sublingual nitroglycerine as needed	Fair – Good	No
Opioid	Codeine Hydrocodone (Hysingla®) Morphine (MS Contin®) Oxycodone (OxyContin®)	Flulike symptoms; insomnia; anxiety; cramps; fatigue; malaise	Mild to Severe	**Management** • Taper over 2 to 3 weeks if severe adverse effects, overdose, or with abuse • Taper by ≤ 10% of original dose per week	Good	No
Proton Pump Inhibitors	Esomeprazole, Lansoprazole, Omeprazole, Pantoprazole	Rebound Acid Secretion (leading to ingestion, heartburn, and reguritation)	Mild to Moderate	**Risk factor** • Continuous therapy > 6 months **Management** • ↓ dose 50% every week, or change from twice daily → once daily, or change from daily use to alternate days	Excellent	No
Skeletal Muscle Relaxants	Baclofen (Lioresal®)	Altered mental status, exaggerated rebound spasticity, high fever, hallucination, confusion, insomnia, muscle rigidity (rarely can lead to rhabdomyolysis, multiple organ-system failure, and death with intrathecal administration)	Mild to Severe	**Risk factors** • Pump malfunction or removal, preventable human errors (programming pump/refill errors), patients with spinal cord injuries at T-6 or above, history of withdrawal symptoms **Maintenance** • Taper over at least 1 to 2 weeks or longer	Excellent	

Notes: References available upon request. List may not represent all medications that have negative effects with abrupt discontinuation.

↑ *Classification of discontinuation symptoms & documentation based on the following criteria*
- *Documentation: Excellent = package inserts, clinical trials, case reports/case series, reported & evaluated frequently in clinical literature; Good = package inserts, clinical trials, case reports/case series, reported & evaluated minimally in clinical literature; Fair = package inserts, case reports/case series, reported & evaluated minimally in clinical literature.*
- *Discontinuation symptom severity: Severe = potentially life threatening with abrupt stopping; Moderate = bothersome, slightly less severe & non-life threatening symptoms; Mild = less severe symptoms but withdrawal reaction present.*

FASTHUG-MAIDENS: Approach to Identifying Drug-Related Problems (DRPs) & Aspects of Critical Care for Intensive Care Units (ICU) Pharmacists

SIDE 1 – FASTHUG

Letter	Area of Care	Role	Examples
F	Feeding	• Discuss feeding route needs. • Medication route changes. • Monitor electrolytes. • Suggest alterations to feeding/supplementation based upon lab results.	• Oral preferred before enteral nutrition before parenteral nutrition • Consider formulation challenges (e.g., crushing medications) • PO (oral) to IV (intravenous) or IV to PO conversions
A	Analgesia	• Assess pain using a pain scale. • Adequate analgesic but not excessive. • Avoid excessive analgesia to minimize respiratory depression. • Opioids + bowel regimen.	• Pain scales: Wong-Baker FACES/Visual Analog Scale/Brief Pain Inventory • Monitor other ways to assess pain in ICU: grimacing; ↑BP; tachycardia • Side effects to consider: respiratory depression, constipation, hypotension, hallucinations & rash
S	Sedation	• Consider non-opioids first (e.g., acetaminophen). • Initiate, discontinue, adjust doses of sedative medications. • Assess sedation as a continuous infusion, intermittent dosing, & as needed. • Avoid excessive sedation to minimize risk of venous thrombosis, intestinal dysmotility	• MV is uncomfortable. • Monitor for: Propofol Infusion Syndrome (PRIS) = cardiac/renal failure & rhabdomylosis, & hypertriglyceridemia • Short-term sedation: dexmedetomidine, propofol vs. Long-term sedation: midazolam, lorazepam • Sedation scales: Richmond Agitation-Sedation Scale (RASS), Riker Sedation-Agitation Scale (SAS)
T	Thromboembolic prophylaxis	• Initiate in almost all patients, unless presence of intracranial or active gastrointestinal bleeding or planned procedure	• LMWH, UFH, compression devices, intravascular filters • Consider mechanical regimens (e.g., sequential compression device [SCD], graduated compression stockings [GCS]).
H	Head of bed elevation; Hyperdelirium & Hypodelirium	• Minimize risk of aspiration pneumonia. • Assess using tools such as Intensive Care Delirium Screening Checklist or Confusion Assessment Method for the ICU.	• Head of bed inclined at 45° to ↓ gastroesophageal reflex in mechanically ventilated patients & nosocomial pneumonia, unless CI (*threatened cerebral perfusion pressure or intracranial hypertension*) ○ ↓ risk of aspiration • For hyper/hypo delirium: supportive & environmental measures, remove/reduce drug-related causes, may consider antipsychotics (e.g., haloperidol, quetiapine).
U	Ulcer (stress) prophylaxis	• Initiate in mechanically ventilated patients • Also indicated for populations at ↑ risk of developing stress ulcers including mechanically ventilated > 48 hours, platelets < 50,000 or INR >1.5, on steroids, history of ulcers, fasting state (i.e., nothing by mouth [NPO]) • Reassess whether prophylactic agent can be discontinued daily	• Add for the duration of hospital stay: histamine receptor antagonists, proton pump inhibitors • Consider discontinuation of stress ulcer prophylaxis at time of discharge.
G	Glycemic control	• Select most appropriate insulin regimens or oral hypoglycemic drugs. • Identify drug-related causes such as glucocorticoids, propofol, atypical antipsychotics. • Achieve goal blood sugar of < 180 mg/dL.	• Consider dosing alterations: insulin drip, basal-glargine, bolus-aspart

Notes: BP = blood pressure; MV = mechanical ventilation; LMWH = Low Molecular Weight Heparin; UFH = Unfractionated Heparin; CI = contraindication.
Based upon: Vincent JM. Give your patient a fast hug (at least) once a day. Crit Care Med 2005;33(6):1225-1229 & Mabasa VH, Malyuk DL, Weatherby EM, Chan A. A Standardized, Structured Approach to Identifying Drug-Related Problems in the Intensive Care Unit: FASTHUG-MAIDENS. CJHP 2011;64(5):366-369.

FASTHUG-MAIDENS: Approach to Identifying Drug-Related Problems (DRPs) & Aspects of Critical Care for Intensive Care Units (ICU) Pharmacists *(continued)*

SIDE 2 — MAIDENS

Letter	Area of Care	Role	Examples
M	Medication reconciliation	• Review medications patient was receiving prior to admission. • Decide which drugs need to be restarted. • Assess medications upon admission, transfer, before discharge. • Identify discontinued medications for high risk of withdrawal symptoms (benzodiazepines, selective serotonin reuptake inhibitors).	• Ask patient "What medications are you currently using" & "How are you taking those medications?" & "Where are those medications filled?" • Ask patient about use of OTC products, such as aspirin, vitamins, pain relievers.
A	Antibiotics/ Anti-infectives	• Selecting optimal antimicrobial agent & de-escalating treatment. • Therapeutic drug monitoring. • Identify appropriate duration of therapy when possible.	• If patient presents with sepsis or septic shock, start broad spectrum antibiotics. Once cultures/susceptibilities are available, modify therapy.
I	Indication for meds	• Review all regularly scheduled & as-needed medications daily. • Any medication that is no longer indicated should be discontinued.	• Identify indication for every medication on the medication list using PMH & HPI (e.g., antihypertensives for high BP)
D	Drug Dosing	• Suggest dose adjustments based on renal & hepatic function. • Therapeutic drug monitoring.	• Monitor CrCl & SCr, eGFR, urine output for kidney function; AST, ALT, albumin, bilirubin for liver function; & adjust dose as needed.
E	Electrolytes/ hematology/other laboratory results	• Monitor patients for drug-related causes of abnormalities in electrolytes, hematology results, or laboratory values & discuss treatment alternatives.	• Refer to Electrolytes & Minerals Card in the Peripheral Brain.
N	No drug interaction/ allergies/ duplications/ADRs	• Identify clinically important potential & actual drug-drug, drug-food, drug-laboratory interactions. • Review allergies at every admission.	• Common drugs to monitor for drug interactions/ADRs: Anticoagulants (e.g., warfarin), sedatives (e.g., midazolam), calcineurin inhibitors (e.g., tacrolimus, cyclosporine), macrolides (e.g., clarithromycin)
S	Stop dates	• Discuss appropriate duration of medications with other members of the health care team.	• Antimicrobial agents, glucocorticoids, opioid infusions

Notes: ADRs = adverse drug reactions; OTC = over-the-counter; PMH = past medical history; HPI = history of present illness; BP = blood pressure; CrCl = creatinine clearance; SCr = serum creatinine; eGFR = glomerular filtration rate; AST = aspartate aminotransferase; ALT = alanine aminotransferase.
Based upon: Mabasa VH, Malyuk DL, Weatherby EM, Chan A. A Standardized, Structured Approach to Identifying Drug-Related Problems in the Intensive Care Unit: FASTHUG-MAIDENS. CJHP 2011;64(5):366-369.

Pharmacy Mnemonics and Memory Aids: Dosing/Drug Names and Interactions

DOSING/DRUG NAMES	
AC/PC	A: A comes before P → before meals; P: Post → post meals
Statin Potency (High to Low): RASP-LF	**R**osuvastatin; **A**torvastatin; **S**imvastatin; **P**ravastatin; **L**ovastatin; **F**luvastatin
Beta 1 and Beta 2	1 Heart → Beta 1 on the heart; 2 Lungs → Beta 2 in the lungs
Opioids: Mu Receptor Effects: MD CARES	**M**iosis; **D**ependency; **C**onstipation; **A**nalgesics; **R**espiratory depression; **E**uphoria; **S**edation
DRUG INTERACTIONS	
Warfarin Interactions: ACADEMIC FACS	**A**miodarone; **C**iprofloxacin/levofloxacin; **A**spirin; **D**icloxacillin; **E**rythromycin (macrolide); **M**etronidazole (azole antifungals); **I**ndomethacin; **C**lofibrates; **F**ibrates; **A**llopurinol; **C**YP 2C9 inducers/inhibitors; **S**tatins
CYP-450 Enzyme Inhibitors: BIG FACES.COM	**B**upropion; **I**traconazole/ketoconazole/fluconazole; **G**emfibrozil; **F**luoxetine/fluvoxamine; **A**miodarone; **C**iprofloxacin; **E**rythromycin/clarithromycin; **S**ulfamethoxazole trimethoprim; **C**lopidogrel; **O**meprazole/esomeprazole; **M**etronidazole
CYP-450 Enzyme Inducers: PS PORCS	**P**henytoin; **S**moking; **P**henobarbital; **O**xcarbazepine; **R**ifampin; **C**arbamazepine; **S**t. John's Wort
Simvastatin Increased Serum Levels: ADIE	**A**miodarone; **D**iltiazem/verapamil; **I**traconazole; **E**rythromycin/clarithromycin

SIDE EFFECTS/CONTRAINDICATIONS	
ACE Inhibitors: CAPTOPRIL	**C**ough; **A**ngioedema; **P**roteinuria/potassium excess; **T**aste changes; **O**rthostatic hypotension; **P**regnancy contraindication/pancreatitis; **R**enal failure/rash; **I**ndomethacin inhibitor; **L**eukopenia/liver toxicity
Steroid: BECLOMETHASONE	**B**uffalo hump; **E**asy bruising; **C**ataracts; **L**arger appetite; **O**besity; **M**oonface; **E**motional changes (instability, euphoria); **T**hin arms and face; **H**yperglycemia/hypertension/hirsutism; **A**septic necrosis; **S**kin (e.g., striae, thinning, bruising with topical preparations); **O**steoporosis; **N**egative nitrogen balance; **E**xtended wound healing
Morphine: MORPHINES	**M**iosis; **O**rthostatic hypotension; **R**espiratory depression; **P**neumonia; **H**istamine release/hormone changes; **I**nfrequency (constipation/urination); **N**ausea; **E**mesis; **S**edation
Increased Potassium (K+) Levels: K-BANK	**K**+ sparing diuretics/supplements; **B**eta blockers; **A**ngiotensin-converting enzyme inhibitors (ACEI)/angiotensin receptor blockers (ARBs): **N**onsteroidal anti-inflammatory drugs (NSAIDs); **K**idney disease
Systemic Corticosteroid Side Effects: CORTICOSTEROIDS	**C**ushing's syndrome; **O**steoporosis; **R**etardation of growth; **T**hin skin/easy bruising; **I**mmunosuppression; **C**ataracts/glaucoma; **O**h-edema; **S**uppression of HPA Axis; **T**eratogenic; **E**motional disturbance; **R**ise in blood pressure; **O**besity; **I**ncreased hair growth (i.e., hirsutism); **D**iabetes mellitus; **S**triae
Decongestants Should Be Avoided: THE DH	**T**hyroid; **H**ypertension; **E**nlarged prostate; **D**iabetes; **H**eart disease
Avoid Use of Antihistamines: AGE	**A**sthma; **G**laucoma; **E**nlarged prostate
Side Effects of Valproate: VALPROATE	**V**omiting; **A**lopecia; **L**iver toxicity; **P**ancreatitis/pancytopenia; **R**etention of fats (weight gain); **O**h - edema; **A**norexia; **T**remor; **E**nzyme inhibitor

Diversity, Equity, Inclusion, Accessibility, Bias, and Cultural Awareness

Definitions

Pharmacists treat diverse populations, and valuing equity and inclusion is vital for effectively engaging and caring for these patients. Pharmacists must recognize connections among health disparities, social determinants of health, and systemic racism.

Diversity	Diversity refers to all aspects of human difference, including, but not limited to, social identities, social group differences, race, ethnicity, creed, color, sex, gender, gender identity, sexual identity, socioeconomic status, language, culture, national origin, religion/spirituality, age, (dis)ability, military/veteran status, political perspective, and associational preference.

EXAMPLES OF DIVERSITY

Culture • Religion/Spirituality • Socioeconomic Status • Color • National Origin • Life Experience • Ethnicity • Geographic Location • Ability • Education • Language • Gender Identity • Age

Prepared by Janan Sarwar and Jeanine Abrons

Diversity, Equity, Inclusion, Accessibility, Bias, and Cultural Awareness *(continued)*

Equity	- Equity refers to fair and just practices and policies that ensure all community members can thrive.
	- Equity is different from equality:
	  - Equality implies treating everyone as if their experiences were the same.
	  - Equity implies acknowledging and addressing structural inequalities (e.g., historic/current) that advance or disadvantage others.
	- Equal treatment results in equity only if everyone starts with equal access to opportunities.
	
	Equality
	The assumption is that everyone benefits from the same support, which is considered to be equal treatment.
	
	Equity
	Everyone gets the support that they individually need, which facilitates equity.
	
	Justice
	The cause(s) of inequity was addressed. The systematic barrier has been removed.

Accessibility	- Accessibility involves ensuring equitable access to everyone along the continuum of human ability and experience. - Communities should design, construct, and develop facilities, programs, and services that include all individuals.
Inclusion	- Inclusion refers to communities where all members are and feel respected, have a sense of belonging, and are able to participate/achieve their potential. - While diversity is essential, it is not sufficient. A community can be both diverse/non-inclusive. - Creating and sustaining inclusive environments is important for successful patient care.

Prepared by Janan Sarwar and Jeanine Abrons

Diversity, Equity, Inclusion, Accessibility, Bias, and Cultural Awareness *(continued)*

Pharmacists' Roles and Responsibilities in Fostering Diversity, Equity, Inclusion, and Accessibility

> *Diversity is about being invited to the party. Inclusion is being part of the party planning committee, choosing the music, and dancing at the party.*
> —Vernā Myers

Why: Pharmacist Roles and Responsibilities

"Truly understanding people's differences and cultures can be a vital part of providing patient care... Obstacles to health can lead to health disparities, which stem from characteristics historically linked to discrimination or exclusion such as race or ethnicity, religion, socioeconomic status, gender, mental health, sexual orientation, or geographic background. Ideally, when health providers recognize cultural differences and work to minimize health disparities, they can achieve health equity."[4]

Vibhuti Arya and colleagues, including president of APhA Sandra Leal, stated: "Systemic racism is a public health emergency and disproportionately impacts communities of color, specifically black Americans. Pharmacists took an oath to protect the welfare of humanity and protect our patients. As such, to practice truly patient-centered care, pharmacists must recognize racism as a root cause of social determinants of health and use their practice."[5]

Definitions

Type of Bias	Description
Confirmation Bias	Tendency to seek out information that supports something you already believe.
Implicit Bias	Perceptions of other cultures as being abnormal or outlying based on a comparison to one's own culture, causing the creation of attitudes or stereotypes that affect or influence decisions in an unconscious way.
Selection Bias	The way individuals notice something more when something has happened to enhance our awareness, making us more observant of subsequent similar things.

Want to become aware of your potential bias? For additional types of biases, please refer to the URL: https://implicit.harvard.edu/implicit/takeatest.html.

Prepared by Janan Sarwar and Jeanine Abrons.

Diversity, Equity, Inclusion, Accessibility, Bias, and Cultural Awareness *(continued)*

Key Terms

Term	Definition
Microagression	Microagressions are verbal, behavioral, or environmental indignities that can be intentional or unintentional and can communicate hostile, derogatory, or harmful prejudicial slights and insults toward culturally marginalized groups.
LGBTQIA	Terms and definitions associated with the LGBTQIA community are evolving. For examples of important definitions please refer to the UC Davis LGBTQIA Resource Center at: https://lgbtqia.ucdavis.edu/educated/glossary
Identity	• Identity is the identifying labels anyone uses to represent themselves; It can also be a system of identifying labels associated with social groups. • Identity gives a sense of belonging to the social world based on similarities within a group.
Intersectionality	• Oxford dictionary defines intersectionality as the interconnected nature of social categories such as race, class and gender, regarded as creating overlapping and interdependent systems of discrimination or disadvantage. • People hold multiple identities and life experiences. • For further information on the impacts to medicine read: Eckstrand KL, Eliason J, St. Cloud T, Potter J. The Priority of Intersectionality in Academic Medicine, *Academic Medicine*, 2016. 91(7): 904–907.
Power Dynamics	• Power is defined as a person's ability to have influence and control. • Power dynamics are how power affects a relationship. Power affects all aspects of our lives and is not inherently negative. For example, parents may influence their children to keep them from harm. If power is abused, it has the capacity to do great harm and can result in oppression or disadvantage to the individual or group with less power.
Privilege	• Privilege is the personal, interpersonal, cultural, and institutional levels that gives advantages, favors, and benefits to members of dominant groups at the expense of members of a less dominant group.

Prepared by Janan Sarwar and Jeanine Abrons

Diversity, Equity, Inclusion, Accessibility, Bias, and Cultural Awareness *(continued)*

Steps in Addressing Your Own Implicit Biases

Consider your own identities:[7]
What is my race, religion, ethnicity, socioeconomic status, gender, sex, sexual orientation, national origin, first language, physical/emotional/developmental (dis)ability, age, and religion or spiritual affiliation?

What identity do you think about most often?	What identities do you think about least often?	What are your identities you want to learn more about?
What identity has the strongest effect on how you perceive yourself?		What identity has the strongest effect on how you perceive others?

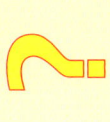

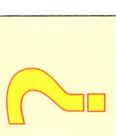

Combat your own implicit biases:[8]

I	M	P	L	I	C	I	T
Introspection	Mindfulness	Perspective Taking	Learn to Slow Down	Individuals	Check Your Messaging	Institutionalize Fairness	Take Two
Explore and identify your biases.	Practice ways to become more mindful.	Consider experiences from the perspectives of others.	Pause and reflect on biases to avoid reflexive actions.	Evaluate based on their own characteristics—don't stereotype.	Embrace evidence-based statements that reduce implicit bias.	Promote procedural change that moves to the socially accountable pharmacy with a goal of health equity.	Practice cultural humility and self-reflection and address power imbalances.

Prepared by Janan Sarwar and Jeanine Abrons

Diversity, Equity, Inclusion, Accessibility, Bias, and Cultural Awareness *(continued)*

SOCIAL DETERMINANTS OF HEALTH & CULTURAL HUMILITY

How to Support Patients with Different Identities and Cultures

Learn the Social Determinants of Health:[9,10]

Economic Stability	Neighborhood and Physical (Build) Environment	Education	Food	Community and Social Context	Health Care Systems
• Employment options • Job benefits (e.g., paid leave, parental leave, health insurance) • Income • Expenses • Debt • Medical bills • Support • Health-related policies	• Housing • Transportation • Safety • Parks • Greenspace • Playgrounds • Walkability • Zip code/geography	• Literacy • Language • Early childhood education • Vocational training • Higher education • Continuing education • Links to working conditions/number of employment options	• Hunger • Access to healthy options • Cost of healthy options • Ability to follow the recommended diet	• Social integration • Support systems • Community engagement • Discrimination • Stress • Availability of support resources • Interpreter availability	• Health coverage • Linguistic and cultural competency • Quality of care • Wait times • The proximity of the nearest pharmacy • Telepharmacy availability • Availability of basic/specialty pharmacy services

Health Outcomes:
Mortality, morbidity, life expectancy, health care expenditures, health status, functional limitations

More visible — above the surface

Iceberg Analogy

UNIVERSAL
• Cultural artifacts/systems
• Cultural values/assumptions

PERSONAL
• The Individual

Takes diving deeper to uncover

CULTURAL

An iceberg is a metaphor for culture (originating from Edward Hall, 1976), which implies that the visible elements of culture provide a surface level of understanding. Deeper observations will uncover additional ideas, beliefs, and attitudes under the surface. This results in a deeper understanding of a culture or individual.

O APhA

146

Diversity, Equity, Inclusion, Accessibility, Bias, and Cultural Awareness *(continued)*

Suggested Steps to Continue Your Exploration of DEIA Based on Your Own Journey

If you are new to Diversity, Equity, Inclusion, and Accessibility (DEIA) Work:

- Learn the language—how diversity, equity, and inclusion are defined.
- Explore trainings or information available from your organization or professional pharmacy organizations such as APhA. To get started, check out additional resources available on PharmacyLibrary.com.
- Some fundamental concepts may include but are not be limited to microaggressions, identity, intersectionality, power dynamics, privilege, and implicit bias.
- Look for ways to impact social determinants of health in your pharmacy.
- Consider where you may have implicit bias and work to address this bias.

If you are ready to learn more about DEIA Work:

- Learn about systemic structures that cause inequities in health care.
- Support marginalized or underserved groups.
- Advocate for and implement policy changes that impact diversity, equity, and inclusion work.
- Explore different social identities: age; first-generation; ability; ethnicity; gender identities; race; religion/spirituality; sex assigned at birth; sexual orientation; socioeconomic status.

If you are leading/want to lead in DEIA Work:

- Foster social awareness.
- Reveal blind spots in your organization/practice and take action to resolve or overcome problems.
- Listen to understand. Use your active listening skills.
- Invite in information from different sources/perspectives.
- Be a potential ally.
- Recognize people as being at different places in their continuum or journey in learning about DEI. Identify where people are at and create safe spaces to have dialogue and engagement.
- There is no finish line in DEI—keep working, keep reflecting, keep growing, and keep improving.

Prepared by Janan Sarwar and Jeanine Abrons

Diversity, Equity, Inclusion, Accessibility, Bias, and Cultural Awareness *(continued)*

Want to know more about diversity, equity, and inclusion as a pharmacist?

Here are a few valuable resources to get you started.

The Centers for Disease Control and Prevention:
This is a go-to reference for information related to the social determinants of health and health disparities. You can also find information linked to the "Healthy People 2030" report.
- Centers for Disease Control and Prevention. Health Disparities and Inequalities Report.
  - *https://www.cdc.gov/minorityhealth/CHDIReport.html.* Accessed November 2021.
- Centers for Disease Control and Prevention. Social Determinants of Health.
  - *https://www.cdc.gov/nchhstp/socialdeterminants/index.html*
  - *https://www.cdc.gov/socialdeterminants/index.htm*

Health.gov:
Look here to find connections between health disparities and diversity, equity, and inclusion work.
- *https://health.gov/healthypeople/tools-action/use-healthy-people-2030-your-work.* Accessed November 2021.

American Association of Colleges of Pharmacy:
- Find resources that are shared with faculty/staff at colleges of pharmacy to further diversity, equity, and inclusion within our profession.
  - American Association of Colleges of Pharmacy. Diversity, Equity, Inclusion and Antiracism Resources. *https://www.aacp.org/deia.* Accessed November 2021.

Other Professions:
As pharmacists, we can look at what other related health professions are doing related to this work. This could include public health, nursing, dentistry, and medicine, as examples.
- American Public Health Association. Equity Diversity Inclusion. Action Toolkit for Organizations. *https://www.apha.org/-/media/files/pdf/affiliates/equity_toolkit.ashx.* Accessed November 2021.
- American Association of Medical Colleges (AAMC). Equity, Diversity, and Inclusion. *https://www.aamc.org/what-we-do/equity-diversity-inclusion.* Accessed November 2021.

Hiring/Letter-Writing Resources:
- Start thinking about how biases enter our professional communications and hiring practices. You can work to put systems in place that help one to be mindful of influences. Implicit biases tend to be even more present when we are under time constraints and stress. Put in structure to make sure these don't influence your decisions.
  - Gender Decoder. Finder Gender Biases in Writing. *https://gender-decoder.katmatfield.com/.* Accessed November 2021.
  - Implicit Bias in Hiring. *https://ucnet.universityofcalifornia.edu/working-at-uc/your-career/talent-management/_files/implicit-bias/Managing_Implicit_Bias_in_the_Hiring_Process_Quick_Reference_Guide.pdf.* Accessed November 2021.
  - Forbes.com. Inclusive Hiring: How to Address Bias in the Recruiting Process. *https://www.forbes.com/sites/forbesbusinesscouncil/2020/10/29/inclusive-hiring-how-to-address-bias-in-the-recruiting-process/?sh=1a8ae375291a.* Accessed November 2021.

Self-Exploration:
Diversity, equity, and inclusion work requires self-examination. Start to know your own biases by taking this insightful test from Harvard University.
- Harvard University. Project Implicit. *https://implicit.harvard.edu/implicit/takeatest.html.* Accessed November 2021.

Prepared by Janan Sarwar and Jeanine Abrons

Herbal and Botanical Therapies

Herbal Therapy Quick Definition: Any plant used internally or externally to treat &/or maintain health.[1]

Common Challenges/Realities of Herbal Medicine:
- Herbal medicine use is common throughout the world. An estimated 80% of the world population lives in locations that rely on herbal therapies.[2,3]
- Consider a patient's belief in use of herbal therapies. Patients may continue to use these options but not inform prescribers of use if negative judgment (or bias against herbs) appears to be present. As a result, distrust, possible interactions & negative outcomes may occur.
- Herbal or botanical medicine is a part of integrative practice that combines both conventional & complementary medicine for which there is evidence on safety & effectiveness.

Goal of Use:
- To help patients integrate herbal therapies with other medications/treatments to support cultural/health beliefs as effectively and safely as possible.
- To suggest resources to providers to enhance knowledge on approaches to herbal or botanical therapies.
- To encourage discussions with patients about benefits & risk of herbal or botanical therapies to enhance ability to create effective integrative approaches.
- To encourage discussion to promote a greater awareness of a complete medication list (or treatments) used by patients.

Warnings/Precautions:
- Herbal therapies or botanical medicine have the potential to create additional risks in special populations (e.g., older adults, pregnant & pediatric populations, those with kidney disease). Use with increased caution.
- Multiple plants may share a common name that may not be widely known. Take additional steps to ensure appropriate understanding. For example, seeing the term "ginseng" may include a number of herbs (i.e., Asian or American ginseng). Record scientific names when possible to reduce the likelihood for error in transferring information.
- Patients & pharmacist should consider obtaining specific references that include scientific & common plant names as well as images to help reduce errors in identifying herbal therapies used by patients.

Enhance Your Knowledge—Things to Learn About Common Herbal Therapies or Botanical Medicine:
- Typical uses &/or benefits
- Proven/potential interactions
- Known safety & efficacy
- Monitoring of adverse effects
- Quality of formulation

Herbal and Botanical Therapies *(continued)*

Recommended Herbal Therapy Resources:

Database	Description of Contents/Use/Link
Natural Medicines *(formerly Natural Standard)*	• Contains use for, safety, effectiveness, dosing & administration, adverse effects, toxicology, drug, herb, food, lab, disease interactions, mechanism of action, & pharmacokinetics.
Micromedex–AltMedDex	• Contains dosing & indications, contraindications/warnings, interactions, adverse effects, & administration
Lexicomp—Natural Products Database	• Contains synonyms, uses & administration, adverse effects, treatment & preparations, & interactions
MedlinePlus*	• https://medlineplus.gov/druginfo/herb_All.html#G
PubMed or NIH Dietary Supplement Subset*	• https://ods.od.nih.gov/Research/PubMed_Dietary_Supplement_Subset.aspx • Designed to limit search results to citations from a broad spectrum of dietary supplements (includes herbals)
Memorial Sloan Kettering "About Herbs"*	• https://www.mskcc.org/cancer-care/diagnosis-treatment/symptom-management/integrative-medicine/herbs/search • Database for the public & healthcare professionals to search common herbs for traditional / proven uses, potential benefits, possible adverse effects, & interactions • Promotes telling professionals herbal therapies used for the reason that an active ingredient can increase or lessen the effects of other medicines
National Center for Complementary & Integrative Health*	• https://nccih.nih.gov/health/herbsataglance.htm • Basic information on specific herbs or botanicals
Cochrane Complementary Medicine*	• https://cam.cochrane.org/ • Promotes systemic reviews of complementary, alternative, & integrative therapies.
Medscape*	• Drug interaction checker includes herbal therapies
Oregon State University Linus Pauling Institute*: Includes hyperlinks and is user friendly	• Consumerlab.com*: Has a free newsletter and can send weekly emails or updates • Hanson and Horn book: Sometimes has editions that have herbal or botanical therapies.

* = Free or open access resource

It is important to look at multiple information sources

References:
1. What are herbal supplements: https://www.hopkinsmedicine.org/health/wellness-and-prevention/herbal-medicine (Accessed 2022)
2. World Health Organization (WHO). WHO Guidelines on Safely Monitoring of Herbal Medicines in Pharmacovigilance Systems. Geneva, Switzerland: WHO.
3. Ekor M. The growing use of herbal medicines: issues relating to adverse reactions & challenges in monitoring safety. Front Pharmcol. 2013;4:177.
4. Milburn MP. Understanding the Convergence of Complementary, Alternative & Conventional Care. https://www.med.unc.edu/phyrehab/pim/files/2018/03/Convergence.text_.pdf (Accessed 2019).
5. Ventola CL. Current Issues regarding Complementary & Alternative Medicine in the United States. 2010;35(8):461–8.
6. Kemper, KJ, Gardiner P, Gobble J, Woods C. Expertise about herbs and dietary among diverse health professionals. BMC complementary and alternative medicine. 2006;6(1):15.
7. Bent S. Herbal medicine in the United States: review of efficacy, safety, and regulation. Journal of general internal medicine. 2008;23(6):854–9.

Herbal and Botanical Therapies *(continued)*

Considerations for Use of Therapies—**Considerations in Weighing Benefits to Risks:**

• Amount/frequency patient consumes/applies	• Desired effects on body/disease state (equivalent to mechanism & indication)*
• Strength/potency of substance	• Timing/duration of effects
• Medication or dietary interactions	• Disease state interactions
• Available sources of knowledge (reputable sources)	• Level of evidence to inform clinical decision making
• Type of preparation	• Consistency/purity of dosage form
• Adverse effects	• Contraindications to use
• Laboratory interactions	• Use in special populations
• Names (scientific/cultural or local/common)	• Potency of plant and active consituents
• Amount used to obtain desired effect**	• Homemade vs. commercial product**

*Effects are often targeted at systems when using botanical therapy. This is contrary to western medicine, which targets a specific ailment. This approach works with your body as opposed to against your body.
**The amount used to obtain desired effects cannot be standardized with homemade products as dosage & strength will vary substantially. Recognize that response is determined by achievement of balance of benefit: Start with the least amount recommended & titrate to the desired effect with a consistent product / source. Monitoring should be frequent.

General Discussion Points with Patients:[6,7]
- Sources of doing your research (how can the patient educate themself on efficacy, contraindications, side effects, drug interactions, & other considerations).
- A common challenge with differences in sourcing therapies is the potential for contamination, misrepresentation, & poor quality of some sources. For both herbal & western medications, when purchasing commercially available products, develop name recognition.
- Discuss individual patient considerations, risks/benefits & alternatives (e.g., comorbidities that may elevate risk, monitoring, cultural beliefs).
- Collaborate: If you don't know something on a therapy, find practitioners who are more well versed.
- Natural versus safe: Herbal medications can also produce effects like allergic reactions or other side effects. Always include every therapy you are pursuing when mentioning medications or treatments to your healthcare provider.
- Consider what the impact is of any treatment to other recommended treatments.

Supplemental Notes to Table:
- The term "insufficient evidence" & possible uses is meant to reflect the presence of lesser amounts of formalized studies of use. However, natural properties/traditional uses may be documented & some studies may exist. For other literature & uses, evaluate on a case by case basis.
- Adverse effects can be explored further for severity/frequency of occurrence or potential use as a therapeutic benefit.

References:
1. Kemper KJ, Gardiner P, Gobble J, Woods C. Expertise about herbs and dietary among diverse health professionals. BMC complementary and alternative medicine. *2006;6(1):15*
2. Bent S. Herbal medicine in the United States: review of efficacy, safety, and regulation. Journal of general internal medicine. *2008;23(6):854–9.*

Herbal and Botanical Medicine

Common Herbs: Effectiveness & Safety: Herbs or Botanical Medicine A to B[1,2]*

Name (Scientific name)	Route & Possibly Safe/Effective	Route & Possibly Safe/Ineffective	Route or Form/Documented Adverse Reactions	Safety Concerns Present/Notes Note: GRAS = generally recognized as safe in food
Aloe (*Aloe vera* & other synonyms)	• **Topical gel:** Acne; burns; herpes simplex virus (HSV); psoriasis • **Oral:** Some dental conditions; gastrointestinal uses; diabetes	• **Topical:** Some dental uses; radiation skin toxicity • **Oral:** HIV/AIDS	• **Aloe gel:** Usually well tolerated; occasional burning, itching, eczema, erythema, dermatitis, & urticaria • **Aloe latex:** Gastrointestinal (GI) (abdominal pain & cramps); diarrhea; ↓ K; albuminuria; hematuria; muscle weakness; weight loss; pigments in intestinal mucosa, prolonged high use: hemorrhagic gastritis; nephritis; renal failure; hepatitis	• **Likely/possibly unsafe:** Aloe taken orally (high doses > 1 g); aloe whole-leaf extract or 'aloe juice' in children or pregnancy & lactation) • Differences exist between aloe gel/latex
Arnica (*Arnica montana, fulgens, sororia, latifolia, & cordifolia*)	• **Topical:** In short-term use on unbroken skin; use in osteoarthritis (twice daily topical use)	• **Topical:** ↓ complications after wisdom tooth extraction	• **With topical:** Allergic reaction with sensitivity to asteraceae/compositae family (e.g., ragweed, marigolds, daisies, etc.) – localized (i.e., irritation, rashes, red spots, allergic eczema; itching; dry skin) • **Oral:** Do not use; ↑ heart rate; palpitations; stomach pain; nausea & vomiting (N/V); diarrhea; muscle weakness; drowsiness; nervousness; headache (HA); shortness of breath	• In food: GRAS • **Insufficient evidence:** ↓ bleeding & bruises; diabetic retinopathy; exercise-induced muscle soreness; postoperative swelling & pain; stroke • **Moderate interaction:** Antiplatelet drugs & anticoagulants
Black Cohosh (*Actaea racemose* & *macrotys*)	• **Oral:** Use up to 6 months; Seems to modestly ↓ symptoms of menopause (e.g., hot flashes) but consider variability in preparations	• **Oral:** Diabetes	• **Oral:** GI upset; rash; HA; dizziness; tiredness; weight gain; heavy legs; cramping; vaginal spotting; hypotension; tiredness; irritability; skin irritation; bleeding; breast tenderness; liver disease; bradycardia; edema; arthralgia & ↑ creatinine phosphokinase (CPK); lactate dehydrogenase (LDH) & high-density lipoprotein (HDL); hormone-sensitive cancers; renal issues; & respiratory distress	• Liver damage in some patients (link to liver failure or autoimmune hepatitis but not conclusive – monitor liver function) • **Unsafe to use in:** Pregnancy (hormonal effects & uterine stimulant → ↑ risk of miscarriage); lactation • **Insufficient evidence:** Breast cancer; cardiovascular disease; infertility; labor induction; migraine HA; osteoarthritis; osteoporosis; rheumatoid arthritis (RA)

Note: Safe use = likely or possibly safe as documented in Natural Standard; safety concerns = likely/possibly unsafe; clinical practitioners must double check for the presence of other medications that can impact safe use or not truly safe; table contains summarized information; for specific studies & > content refer to databases listed above

Herbal and Botanical Medicine *(continued)*

Common Herbs: Effectiveness & Safety: Herbs or Botanical Medicine Bl to Ci[1,2]*

Name *(Scientific name)*	Route & Possibly Safe/Effective	Route & Possibly Safe/Ineffective	Route or Form/Documented Adverse Reactions	Safety Concerns Present/Notes *Note: GRAS = generally recognized as safe in food*
Blessed thistle *(Cnicus benedictus)*	• **Oral:** Usually safe when used at recommended doses for short period of time	• **Oral:** N/A—see notes	• **Oral:** Few adverse reactions but cases of dermatitis, stomach irritation may occur with high doses; increased bleeding risk; eye irritation & nephrotoxicity from chronic indigestion of tannins are reported	• **Insufficient evidence to rate:** Possibly safe for use of loss of appetite & indigestion; as an antidiarrheal, expectorant, antibiotic, & diuretic; for promoting lactation & treating colds/fever • **Unsafe to use in:** Pregnancy; insufficient reliable information with lactation • **Minor interactions:** Antacids; H2-blockers; proton pump inhibitors (PPIs) • **In food:** GRAS
Chamomile (German) *(Matricaria recutita)*	• **Oral:** In medicinal amounts for dyspepsia, diarrhea, & generalized anxiety disorder (GAD)	• **Topical:** Use in Radiation dermatitis	• **Oral:** Hypersensitivity reactions can occur & naphylaxis, nausea, burning in the mouth • **Topical:** Allergic dermatitis, eczema; if used near eyes: irritation	• Avoid confusion with Roman Chamomile • **Insufficient evidence to rate:** eczema; colic; cold; gingivitis; hemorrhoids; insomnia; mucositis; lesions/healing; incontinence; pregnancy; lactation • **Minor interactions:** Cytochrome P450 (CYP) 1A2 substrates • **Moderate interactions:** benzodiazepines; CNS depressants; contraceptives; CYP 2C9/3A4 substrates; estrogens; tamoxifen; warfarin
Cinnamon *(Cinnamomum aromaticum—large list of additional names)*	• **Oral:** For diabetes (↓ blood glucose; total cholesterol (TC); triglycerides (TG); ↑ high density lipoprotein (HDL)	• **Oral:** Not applicable (N/A)—see notes	• **Oral:** Usually well tolerated; at high doses: vomiting (conflicting data); concern of hepatic safety (due to coumarin content) • **Topical:** Allergic reaction	• **Insufficient evidence:** Impaired glucose tolerance (pre-diabetes), mosquito repellent; pregnancy & lactation (avoid use) • **Possibly safe:** Topical use; short term; oral use in children • **Unsafe to use in:** High doses & long-term • **Moderate interactions:** Diabetes drugs; cautious use with hepatotoxic drugs

*Note: Safe use = likely or possibly safe as documented in Natural Standard; safety concerns = likely/possibly unsafe; clinical practitioners must double check 'for the presence of other medications that can impact whether or not truly safe; table contains summarized information; for specific studies & > content refer to databases listed above

Herbal and Botanical Medicine (continued)

Common Herbs: Effectiveness & Safety: Herbs or Botanical Medicine Cr to Ea[1,2]*

Name (Scientific name)	Route & Possibly Safe/ Effective	Route & Possibly Safe/Ineffective	Route or Form/Documented Adverse Reactions	Safety Concerns Present/Notes Note: GRAS = generally recognized as safe in food
Cranberry *Vaccinium macrocarpon, oxycoccos, hagerupii, microcarpum, & synonyms)*	• **Oral:** Use in urinary tract infections; use in children	• **Oral:** Use in diabetes	• **Oral:** Usually well tolerated; at high doses: stomach upset & diarrhea; skin redness/ itching; possible ↑ in blood glucose (found in 1 patient); vaginal itching/dryness; thrombocytopenia; concern of hepatotoxicity with high coumarin content	• **Insufficient evidence to rate:** Benign prostatic hyperplasia (BPH); cold/flu; coronary artery disease (CAD); H. pylori; kidney stones; memory; metabolic syndrome; urinary odor • **Minor interactions:** Cytochrome (CYP) P450 2C9 substrates; diclofenac • **Moderate interactions:** Atorvastatin; CYP 3A4 substrates; nifedipine; warfarin
Echinacea *(Echinacea angustifolia, pallida, purpea)*	• **Oral:** Treatment/prevention (conflicting evidence) of common cold, when used short-term	• **Oral/Topical:** N/A—see notes	• **Oral:** Usually well tolerated; gastrointestinal—nausea/ vomiting (N/V); itching, urticaria; leukopenia; hepatic changes; immunologic	• **Insufficient evidence:** Anxiety; atopic dermatitis; exercise performance; gingivitis; herpes simplex virus (HSV); human papilloma virus (HPV); influenza; leukopenia; otitis media; tonsillitis; uveitis; warts • **Minor interactions:** Lopinavir/ritonavir (↑); midazolam (↑ oral availability) • **Moderate interactions:** Caffeine (↑); CYP 1A2 (inhibits) & 3A4 (Varied); etoposide (inhibits metabolism); immunosuppressants; • Other drug interactions severity rated as insignificant

Note: Safe use = likely or possibly safe as documented in Natural Standard; safety concerns = likely/possibly unsafe; clinical practitioners must double check for the presence of other medications that can impact whether or not truly safe; table contains summarized information; for specific studies & > content refer to databases listed above

Herbal and Botanical Medicine (continued)

Common Herbs: Effectiveness & Safety: Herbs or Botanical Medicine El to Ev[1,2]*

Name (*Scientific name*)	Route & Possibly Safe/Effective	Route & Possibly Safe/Ineffective	Route or Form/Documented Adverse Reactions	Safety Concerns Present/Notes *Note: GRAS = generally recognized as safe in food*
Elderberry (*Sambucus nigra*)	• **Oral:** Constipation; ↓ flu-like symptoms	• **Oral:** Not applicable (N/A)—see notes	• **Oral:** Usually well tolerated; N/V when used with echinacea; allergic reaction; some effects associated with raw fruit (e.g., dizziness; numbness; stupor)	• **Insufficient evidence:** Cardiovascular disease; common cold; hyperlipidemia • **Minor interactions:** Cytochrome P450 (CYP) 3A4 substrates • **Moderate interactions:** mmunosuppressants
Evening primrose (*Oenothera biennis*)	• **Oral:** Menopause	• **Oral:** Asthma; attention deficit-hyperactivity disorder; pre-eclampsia	• **Oral:** Usually well tolerated; transient gastrointestinal (GI) effects most common (ab pain; distention; fullness; N/V; diarrhea; dyspepsia; flatulence); skin rash; acne; ↓ platelet aggregation; dizziness; headache (HA); weight gain	• **Insufficient evidence:** A:opic dermatitis; biliary disorders; chronic fatigue syndrome (CFS); diabetic neuropathy; dry eyes; dyslexia; dyspraxia; Hepatitis B; hyperlipidemia; ichthyosis; infant development; liver cancer; mastalgia; mencpausal symptoms; obesity; parturition; psoriasis; premenstrual syndrome; arthritis; Raynaud's; schizophrenia; Sjogren's; tardive dyskinesia; ulcerative colitis • **Moderate interactions:** Anesthesia; anticoagulants/antiplatelets; lopinavir/ritonavir; phenothiazines • Other drug interactions severity rated as insignificant

*Note: Safe use = likely or possibly safe as documented in Natural Standard; safety concerns = likely/possibly unsafe; clinical practitioners must double check for the presence of other medications that can impact whether or not truly safe; table contains summarized information; for specific studies & > content refer to databases listed above

Herbal and Botanical Medicine *(continued)*

Common Herbs: Effectiveness & Safety: Herbs or Botanical Medicine Fe[1,2]*

Name *(Scientific name)*	Route & Possibly Safe/Effective	Route & Possibly Safe/Ineffective	Route or Form/Documented Adverse Reactions	Safety Concerns Present/Notes *Note: GRAS = generally recognized as safe in food*
Fenugreek *(Trigonella foenum-graecum)*	• **Oral:** Diabetes; dysmenorrhea; sexual dysfunction • Possibly safe when used in medicinal amounts up to 6 months	• **Oral:** None applicable (N/A)—see notes	• **Oral:** Mild GI effects (diarrhea); dyspepsia; abdominal distention; nausea; flatulence); allergic reactions; dizziness; HA • **Topical/Inhalation:** Allergic reactions	• **Insufficient evidence:** Exercise function; gastroesophageal reflux disease (GERD); hyperlipidemia; lactation; infertility; obesity; Parkinson's; polycystic ovary syndrome (PCOS) • **Unsafe to use in:** Pregnancy; possibly in children • **Moderate interactions:** Anticoagulants/antiplatelets; antidiabetic drugs; theophylline; warfarin
Feverfew *(Tanacetum parthenium)*	• **Oral:** When used appropriately, short term (4-months) for migraines	• **Oral:** Rheumatoid arthritis (RA)	• **Oral:** Usually well tolerated; may be better tolerated than some conventional migraine drugs; may cause palpitations; skin rash; allergic dermatitis; GI effects (heartburn; nausea; diarrhea; constipation; ab pain/bloating; flatulence); joint stiffness; nervousness; insomnia; dizziness; tiredness; menstrual changes; weight gain	• **Insufficient evidence:** Pruritus (itching) • **Unsafe to use in:** Pregnancy; insufficient evidence in lactation; when fresh leaves are chewed • **Moderate interactions:** Anticoagulant/antiplatelet drugs; CYP 2C19, 2C8, 2C9, 2D6, 3A4 substrates

Note: Safe use = likely or possibly safe as documented in Natural Standard; safety concerns = likely/possibly unsafe; clinical practitioners must double check for the presence of other medications that can impact whether or not truly safe; table contains summarized information; for specific studies & > content refer to databases listed above

Herbal and Botanical Medicine (continued)

Common Herbs: Effectiveness & Safety: Herbs or Botanical Medicine Ginger[1,2]* to Gingko[1,2]*

Name (Scientific name)	Route & Possibly Safe/Effective	Route & Possibly Safe/Ineffective	Route or Form/Documented Adverse Reactions	Safety Concerns Present/Notes Note: GRAS = generally recognized as safe in food
Ginger (*Zingiber officinale*)	• **Oral:** Antiretroviral-induced nausea/vomiting (N/V); dysmenorrhea; osteoarthritis; pregnancy-induced N/V	• **Oral:** Exercise-induced muscle soreness; motion sickness	• **Oral:** Usually well tolerated at typical doses; high doses (> 5 grams per day) increase side effects & ↑ tolerability; mild arrhythmia in one patient; rash/hives; bruising; flushing; nausea; belching; vomiting; ab discomfort; heartburn; diarrhea; constipation; ↑ menstrual bleeding; sedation; drowsiness; dizziness; conjunctivitis	• **Insufficient evidence:** Acute respiratory distress syndrome (ARDS); chemotherapy and iced N/V; chronic obstructive pulmonary disease (COPD); dyspepsia; hangover; hyperlipidemia; hypertension; irritable bowel; joint pain; migraine; parturition; postoperative N/V & recovery; swallowing dysfunction; liver damage • **Possibly safe to use in:** Pregnancy; children; insufficient evidence in lactation • **Minor interactions:** Antidiabetic drugs; calcium channel blockers; cyclosporine; metronidazole • **Moderate interactions:** Anticoagulants/antiplatelets; phenprocoumon; warfarin; nifedipine
Ginkgo (*Ginkgo biloba*)	• **Oral:** When used appropriately, short term (4 months) for anxiety; dementia; diabetic retinopathy; glaucoma; peripheral vascular disease; premenstrual syndrome (PMS); schizophrenia; tardive dyskinesia; cognitive impairment; sexual dysfunction; chemotherapy complications; hypertension; multiple sclerosis; seasonal affective disorder	• **Oral:** Macular degeneration; hay fever; asthma; attention deficit-hyperactivity disorder; chronic obstructive pulmonary disease; cognitive function; dyslexia; fibromyalgia; hearing loss; migraines; Raynaud's; stroke; vitiligo	• **Oral:** Usually well tolerated in typical doses (leaf extract)—can cause headache (HA), dizziness, palpitations, constipation, & allergic skin reactions • **Topical:** Fruit & pulp can cause severe allergic reactions & mucosal irritation	• Likely safe if used orally & appropriately, but concern exists of toxic & carcinogenic effects seen in animals • Avoid ingestion of crude plant parts • Cross reactivity possible if a lergic to poison ivy/oak/sumac, mango rind, & cashew shell • **Possibly unsafe:** If roasted seed or crude plant is consumed; use in pregnancy; insufficient evidence in lactation • **Likely unsafe:** If fresh seed is used orally • **Possibly safe in:** Children (short-term use) • **Major interactions:** Talinolol • **Moderate interactions:** Alprazolam; anticoagulants/antiplatelets; anticonvulsants; antidepressants; antidiabetic drugs; buspirone; CYP 1A2, 2C19, 2C9, 2D6, 3A4 substrates; efavirenz; fluoxetine; ibuprofen; nonnucleoside reverse transcriptase inhibitors; risperidone; seizure threshold ↓ drugs; simvastatin; warfarin • **Minor interactions:** Hydrochlorothiazide; nifedipine

Note: Safe use = likely or possibly safe as documented in Natural Standard; safety concerns = likely/possibly unsafe; clinical practitioners must double check for the presence of other medications that can impact whether or not truly safe; table contains summarized information; for specific studies & > content refer to databases listed above

Herbal and Botanical Medicine (continued)

Common Herbs: Effectiveness & Safety: Herbs or Botanical Medicine Gi to Ra[1,2]*

Name (Scientific name)	Route & Possibly Safe/Effective	Route & Possibly Safe/Ineffective	Route or Form/Documented Adverse Reactions	Safety Concerns Present/Notes Note: GRAS = generally recognized as safe in food
Ginseng (*Panax ginseng*)	• **Oral:** When used short term; Alzheimer's disease; chronic obstructive pulmonary disease; cognitive function; flu • **Topical:** Short-term use for erectile dysfunction	• **Oral:** Athletic performance	• **Oral:** Usually well tolerated at typical doses; most common = insomnia; less common = mastalgia, vaginal bleeding, amenorrhea, blood pressure changes; edema; ↓ appetite; diarrhea; pruritus; headache; euphoria; mania; controversial = possible estrogenic effects	• **Insufficient evidence:** Breast cancer; bronchitis; common cold; heart failure; fibromyalgia; gallbladder disease; halitosis; hangover; hearing loss; HIV/AIDS; hypertension; prediabetes; male infertility; memory; menopause; wrinkled skin • **Possibly unsafe:** Long-term use (hormone-like effects); use in children & pregnancy; insufficient evidence in lactation • **Moderate interactions:** Anticoagulants/antiplatelet drugs; alcohol; antidiabetic drugs; caffeine; CYP 3A4; estrogens; furosemide; imatinib; insulin; midazolam; monoamine oxidase inhibitors; nifedipine; QT interval-prolonging drugs; raltegravir; stimulants; warfarin • **Minor interactions:** Fexofenadine; CYP 1A1 substrates
Raspberry ketones (*4-(4-Hydroxyphenl) butan-2-one*)	• **Oral:** None applicable (N/A)—see notes	• **Oral:** None applicable (N/A)—see notes	• **Oral:** Shakiness; heart palpitations; stimulant-related side effects	• **Insufficient evidence:** Alopecia areata; androgenic alopecia; weight loss; safety information in general • **Possibly safe to use in:** Pregnancy; insufficient evidence in lactation • **Moderate interactions:** Antidiabetic drugs; stimulants; warfarin; with diabetes (↓ blood sugars)

*Note: Safe use = likely or possibly safe as documented in Natural Standard; safety concerns = likely/possibly unsafe; clinical practitioners must double check for the presence of other medications that can impact whether or not truly safe; table contains summarized information; for specific studies & > content refer to databases listed above

Herbal and Botanical Medicine *(continued)*

Common Herbs: Effectiveness & Safety: Herbs or Botanical Medicine Re to Sa[1,2]*

Name *(Scientific name)*	Route & Possibly Safe/Effective	Route & Possibly Safe/Ineffective	Route or Form/Documented Adverse Reactions	Safety Concerns Present/Notes *Note: GRAS = generally recognized as safe in food*
Red Yeast Rice *(Monscus purpureus)*	• **Oral:** Hyperlipidemia (1 to 5 grams daily) with long-term use; cardiovascular disease	• **Oral:** Hypertension	• **Oral:** Abdominal discomfort; heartburn; fatigue; flatulence; headache (HA); dizziness; elevated liver enzymes; kidney damage; myalgias; muscle spasm; myopathy, rhabdomyolysis; tachycardia; ↑ creatinine kinase; uncommonly = edema; mild rash; anaphylaxis	• **Insufficient evidence:** Cancer; diabetes; metabolic syndrome; nonalcoholic fatty liver disease • **Likely unsafe:** In pregnancy; insufficient evidence in lactation • **Moderate interactions:** Alcohol; cyclosporine; CYP 3A4 inhibitors; gemfibrozil; hepatotoxic drugs; statins; niacin; St. John's wort
Saw Palmetto *(Serenoa repens)*	• **Oral:** Transurethral resection of prostate	• **Oral:** Benign prostatic hyperplasia (BPH)	• **Oral:** Generally mild side effects; Dizziness; HA; nausea/vomiting; constipation; diarrhea; loss of libido; ejaculation disorders; erectile dysfunction; weakness; pain; ↑ bleeding; insomnia; occasional = hypotension, arrhythmias, heart failure, myocardial infarction; worsening acne	• **Insufficient evidence:** Androgenic alopecia; hypotonic bladder; prostate cancer; prostatitis • **Moderate interactions:** Anticoagulant/antiplatelet drugs; contraceptive drugs; estrogens; liver function tests • **Likely unsafe:** In pregnancy & lactation

Note: Safe use = likely or possibly safe as documented in Natural Standard; safety concerns = likely/possibly unsafe; clinical practitioners must double check for the presence of other medications that can impact whether or not truly safe; table contains summarized information; for specific studies & > content refer to databases listed above

Herbal and Botanical Medicine *(continued)*

Common Herbs: Effectiveness & Safety: Herbs or Botanical Medicine St[1,2,3,4]* to Tu[1,2,3,4]*

Name (Scientific name)	Route & Possibly Safe/Effective	Route & Possibly Safe/Ineffective	Route or Form/Documented Adverse Reactions	Safety Concerns Present/Notes *Note: GRAS = generally recognized as safe in food*
St. John's wort (*Hypericum perforatum*)	• **Oral:** Depression; menopausal symptoms; wound healing	• **Oral:** Burning mouth syndrome	• **Oral:** Usually well tolerated at typical doses; vivid dream; restlessness; anxiety; agitation; irritability; gastrointestinal (GI); fatigue; dry mouth; dizziness; headache; rash; hypoglycemia; edema; photodermatitis; menstrual changes; rarely—muscle spasm, tremor or pain	• **Major interactions:** Alprazolam; contraceptive drugs; cyclosporine; CYP 3A4 substrates; digoxin; docetaxel; fenfluramine; imatinib; irinotecan; ketamine; mephenytoin; nonnucleoside reverse transcriptase inhibitors; omeprazole; oxycodone; P-glycoprotein substrates; phenobarbital; pheprocoumon; phenytoin; protease inhibitors; tacrolimus; warfarin • **Moderate interactions:** 5-HT1 agonists; aminolevulinic acid; antidepressants; barbiturates; bupropion; clopidogrel; clozapine; CYP 1A2, 2B6, 2C19, 2C9 substrates; dextromethorphan; fentanyl; fexofenadine; finasteride; gliclazide; statins; indinavir; ivabradine; meperidine; methadone; monoamine oxidase inhibitors; nefazodone; nifedipine; paroxetine; photosensitizing drugs; reserpine; tramadol; verapamil; voriconazole
Turmeric (*Curcuma longa*)	• **Oral:** Hay fever; depression; hyperlipidemia; nonalcoholic fatty liver disease; osteoarthritis; pruritis	• **Oral:** Peptic ulcers; radiation dermatitis	• **Oral:** Skin sensitization problems; bitter taste; generally well tolerated; when taken in large doses, may cause GI problems & heart issues • **Topical:** Contact dermatitis; urticaria; photosensitivity when taken with fluoxetine	• **Insufficient evidence:** Curcuminoid component helps to ↓ inflammation & role in ↓ of heart attacks; ↓ knee pain; ↓ skin irritation; cancers; diabetes; plaque ↓; cognitive ↓; asthma; coronary artery bypass surgery (CABG); metabolic syndrome; arthritis; ulcerative colitis • **Likely unsafe:** Contraindicated in pregnancy & lactation, gallstones, gallbladder obstruction, hyperacidity, ulcers, bile obstruction • **Moderate drug interactions:** Anticoagulants/antiplatelet drugs; antidiabetic drugs; camptothecin; cyclophosphamide; cytochrome P450 (CYP) 3A4 substrate; doxorubicin; estrogens; sulfathalazine; tacrolimus; talinolol • **Minor drug interactions:** CYP 1A1, 1A2 substrate; docetaxel; glyburide; norfloxacin; P-glycoprotein substrates; paclitaxel

1. Pursell, J.J. (2015). *The Herbal Apothecary 100 Medicinal Herbs and How to Use Them.* Therm. Portland, Oregon, Timber
2. Therapeutic Research Center (TRC). *Natural Medicines™.* https://naturalmedicines.therapeuticresearch.com/databases/food,-herbs-supplements (Accessed 2021)
3. National Center for Complementary & Integrative Health: https://nccih.nih.gov/health/herbsataglance.htm (Accessed 2021)
4. Micromedex: https://www.micromedexsolutions.com (Accessed 2021)

Basics of Medical Cannabis

General
Of the many natural medicines, medical cannabis has grown exponentially in popularity over the last decade. The two most active compounds are the phytocannabinoids, tetrahydrocannabinol (THC), and cannabidiol (CBD). The terminology distinguishing Cannabis sativa and Cannabis indica is now less commonly used due to the prevalence of hybridization of plants. Israeli organic chemist and professor Raphael Mechoulam is also known as the "father of cannabis research" and is credited for the isolation and structure elucidation of the active components of the plant.

Timeline of Medical Cannabis Laws in the United States

Year	Law/Description
1937	• The Marijuana Tax Act of 1937 criminalized the recreational use of cannabis. The legislation was the first of many that shaped the country's attitude and perception toward the rise of immigration and the use of the plant.
1972	• Nixon repealed the Marijuana Tax Act and declared marijuana a Schedule I drug, meaning that it had no accepted medical use and had a high potential of abuse, under the Controlled Substance Act.
2018	• The Agricultural Improvement Act of 2018 (also known as the 2018 Farm Bill) was passed, legalizing the use of industrialized hemp under federal law. It mandated that legal hemp-derived CBD products must contain < 0.3% THC.
2020	• As of October, cannabis is legal for medical use in 33 states, the District of Columbia, Guam, and Puerto Rico, with varying restrictions. In states where it is legal for medical use, patients require a specific medical marijuana card. CBD is federally legal; however, cannabis remains a Schedule I controlled substance. In most cases, state jurisdiction overrules federal legislation; for example, Idaho, Nebraska, and South Dakota have deemed CBD illegal regardless of the 2018 Farm Bill.

Sample legality resource: https://disa.com/map-of-marijuana-legality-by-state; https://www.ncsl.org/research/health/state-medical-marijuana-laws.aspx (Accessed 2020)

Regulations related to medical cannabis are made on a state by state basis and are rapidly changing.

Cards by Swathi Varanasi and Jeanine P. Abrons

FDA-Approved Medical Cannabis Products

CBD	THC	Other Products
• Major Cannabinoid* • **Plant-Derived CBD** Cannabidiol (Epidiolex): Descheduled from CV (2020) Dosage Form: Oral solution containing sesame oil Indications: Lennox-Gastaut syndrome (LGS) or Dravet syndrome (DS) in patients 2 years of age and older	• Major Cannabinoid* • **Synthetic THC** Dronabinol (Marinol): CIII (1985) Dosage Form: Oral capsules Indications: CINV**, anorexia associated with weight loss in patients with AIDS Nabilone (Cesamet): CII (1985) Dosage Form: Oral capsules Indication: CINV	• **Plant-Derived Cannabinoids** Nabiximols (Sativex)***: CBD: THC 1:1 ratio Dosage Form: Oromucosal spray Indications: Muscle symptoms and spasms associated with multiple sclerosis (MS)

*Referred to as major cannabinoid because it is found at high concentrations in cannabis plant (in contrast to minor cannabinoids)

**CINV = Chemotherapy-induced nausea/vomiting

***As of 2019, nabiximols was licensed in 29 countries across the world. They were allowed in countries like Spain and the UK, where medical cannabis remains an illegal substance, and is in Phase II and III clinical trials worldwide.

Minor Cannabinoids

CBG   CBG-A   THC-A   THC-V   CBC   CBC-A   CBC-V   CBD-A   CBD-V   CBN

Methods of Administration

Cannabis can be purchased in many formulations (see below). Product legality standards/availability are highly state-specific.

- Smoking
- Vaporizing
- Edible/Gummies
- Capsules/Tablets
- Topicals/Transdermals
- Syrups
- Tinctures
- Sprays
- Oils
- Suppositories

Possible Uses of Medical Cannabis

Possible ADULT Uses

• Anxiety	• Autism	• Appetite	• Cachexia	• CINV*
• Crohn's disease	• Dementia	• Epilepsy	• Fibromyalgia	• Glaucoma
• HIV-related wasting	• Migraine	• Multiple sclerosis	• Muscle spasms	• Nausea
• Pain	• Parkinson's disease	• Rheumatoid arthritis	• Ulcerative colitis	

*Chemotherapy-induced nausea and vomiting

Possible PEDIATRIC Uses

- Acne
- Anxiety
- Chemotherapy-related
- Epilepsy
- Diabetes

Cards by Swathi Varanasi and Jeanine P. Abrons

APhA

Pharmacology Basics of Medical Cannabis

Pharmacology & The Endocannabinoid System
- Cannabis acts on the endocannabinoid system.
- Properties of the endocannabinoid system: linked with a majority of organ/neurotransmitter systems → modulates many bodily processes to achieve the goal of maintaining homeostasis, or balance.
  - ***Two receptors (CB1; CB2); G-protein–coupled receptors located throughout the body***
    - CB1: Primarily found in the central nervous system
    - CB2: More closely associated with immune function
- **Other receptors:** Work directly/indirectly in the endocannabinoid system (e.g., 5HT1A, TRPV1, PPARγ, GPR119, and others).
- **Phytocannabinoids Found in Plants:**
  - THC: CB1 receptor = high affinity → infamous euphoric effects ("feeling high"); CB2 receptor = lower affinity; primarily metabolized by CYP3A4 and 2A9
  - CBD: Modulates the endocannabinoid system, but the exact mechanism is unclear; primarily metabolized by CYP3A4 and 2C19
- **Body's Own Cannabinoids:** Different from the phytocannabinoids
  - Called endocannabinoids; the two discovered are anandamide (AEA) and 2-arachidonoylglycerol (2-AG)
  - Acts on the cannabinoid receptors/non-cannabinoid receptors endocannabinoid tone (i.e., basic system functionality)
  - It has been thought that there is what has been referred to as an entourage effect. This means that all the components in the cannabis plant work in synergy.

Understanding the Complexity:
- Medications may often be viewed as a simple active compound with one molecule–one effect.
- Botanical medicines (e.g., medical cannabis) are more complex.
- As a plant, cannabis has numerous phytocannabinoids, terpenes, and constituents that influence the human body.
- The major phytocannabinoids are metabolized by the CYP450 family of enzymes (see above for specifics).
- Much research on drug interactions with cannabis is completed at much higher doses than your patients will take.

Dosing/Side Effects of Medical Cannabis

Dosing Principles:
- General principle is to start low and go slow and stay low.
- For tinctures—start with a quarter of a pipette. Use for at least two nights/days and then gradually titrate up to the desired effect. Use with consistency initially and then may be adjusted as needed.
- It is recommended that natural medicine and cannabis specialists are involved in the care of patients interested in adding cannabis to a regimen as the range of products and varying concentrations of CBD, THC, and other minor cannabinoids make dosing complicated & highly patient-specific.
- Encourage patients to tell all of their healthcare providers & practitioners about their use of prescription medications, dietary supplements, herbs (including cannabis), homeopathy, & other types of healing modalities.

Possible SIDE EFFECTS:
- Dizziness
- Dry Mouth
- Fatigue

World Health Organization for Cannabis Dependence:
- There is controversy on whether cannabis use can lead to addiction. Authoritative bodies (e.g., WHO) and reference guides such as the DSM-V have statements regarding cannabis use disorder or cannabis use dependence. As of 2020, there is no concrete evidence that supports cannabinoid receptors' direct involvement in addiction. Be careful in labeling a patient as having an addiction & be willing to have an open conversation on reasons for use.

Cards by Swathi Varanasi and Jeanine P. Abrons

Medical Cannabis & Examples of Drug Interactions

Moderate Interactions with Moderate Severity	Moderate Interaction with High Severity
• **Specific Drugs/Classes:** 　○ Anesthesia 　○ Disulfiram • **Cytochrome P450 Inhibitors & Inducers:** 　○ **CYP1A2, CYP2C9, CYP2D6, CYP2E1, CYP3A4**	• **Specific Drugs/Classes:** 　○ Antiplatelet/anticoagulant 　○ Barbiturates 　○ CNS Depressants 　○ P-glycoprotein substrates 　○ Theophylline 　○ Thrombolytics • **Cytochrome P450 Inhibitors & Inducers:** 　○ CYP1A2, CYP2C9, CYP2D6, CYP2E1, CYP3A4

Carbamazepine	Carisoprodol	Cimetidine
Cimetidine	Citalopram	Clopidogrel
Diazepam	Fluconazole	Phenobarbital
Phenytoin	PPIs	Primidone
Rifampin		

PPI = Proton Pump Inhibitors

Carbamazepine	**Clobazam**	Cyclosporine
Fluoxetine	Glucocorticoids	Ketoconazole
Macrolides	Mirtazapine	Ritonavir
St. John's wort	**Tacrolimus**	**Valproic acid**
Verapamil	Voriconazole	**Warfarin**

Drugs in red = absolute contraindications; see below for additional information

- Interactions between medical cannabis & drugs may result in competitive inhibition or induction which may increase or decrease both the drug & the active cannabinoid levels. The amounts of various active cannabinoids can influence the nature of the drug interaction.
- Consider factors such as the dose of the medications, route, frequency and amounts of medical cannabis consumed to determine the level of significance of the drug interaction. **For specific concerns, consult a medical cannabis specialist.**
- <u>**ABSOLUTE CONTRAINDICATIONS:**</u> Valproic acid, clobazam, & warfarin; medications with narrow therapeutic indexes &/or for immunosuppressive conditions. **For concerns with specific drugs, contact a medical cannabis specialist.**

Medical Cannabis: Evidence and Special Populations

Population	Description
Elderly	• Recorded as most-frequent users of cannabis for medical purposes • Review of possible drug–drug interactions is of utmost concern with this population
Opioid Dependence	• An emerging area of use involving consultation with cannabis specialist practitioners who provide tapering regimens to reduce and/or eliminate opioid dependence
Pediatrics	• First plant-derived cannabis therapy approved in 2018 for LGS and DS • Research is limited and therefore the inclusion of a cannabis specialist is highly recommended
Pregnancy & Lactation	• Research is inconclusive regarding the use of cannabis; not recommended at this time
Other	• Patients with bipolar disorder and schizophrenia should be cautioned with consuming high levels of THC as they may experience increased levels of paranoia and psychoactive effects. • Contact a medical cannabis specialist for questions regarding use of cannabis for or during COVID.

Evidence-Based Practice:
- Cannabis research is a relatively new and growing area of focus that is rapidly evolving. For the most up-to-date literature, the pharmacist should consult and review resources provided below.

Cards by Swathi Varanasi and Jeanine P. Abrons

Cannabidiol (CBD): A Naturally Occurring Cannabinoid Found in Cannabis

- Modulates the endocannabinoid system to improve endocannabinoid tone, or the overall system functionality and its relationship with regulating other organ and neurotransmitter systems in the body.
- Studies show CBD as an option for patients for easing anxiety, relieving pain, and modulating the sleep/wake cycle.
- Research is studying the use of CBD for weight loss/obesity, cardiovascular disease, depressed mood, and skin diseases. Unlike THC, CBD doesn't produce the euphoric effects of "feeling high," also known as intoxication.

Evaluating Whether It Is a Good CBD Brand:

- Encourage patients to look for a Certificate of Analysis (COA) as a primary marker of the quality of the product. Manufacturers should either have this information readily posted or be able to produce the documentation quickly.

CBD Product Terminology: Isolate vs. Broad-Spectrum vs. Full Spectrum

- When deciding between the three types, CBD Isolate, Broad Spectrum, or Full Spectrum, many cannabis providers are in favor of broad spectrum or full spectrum given the synergistic or entourage effect. By incorporating more than one cannabinoid, the patient could achieve desired effects with a lower dose. Traditionally, in Aryuveda and Traditional Chinese Medicine, the entire cannabis plant has been used, which is similar to broad or full spectrum.

Term	Description
CBD Isolate	Product that contains only CBD
Broad Spectrum	The product contains CBD, minor cannabinoids, and terpenes, but NO THC
Full Spectrum	The product contains CBD, minor cannabinoids, terpenes, and less than 0.3% THC

The Emerging Role for Pharmacists:

- A pharmacist's role depends upon state and local regulations. In some states, a requirement exists that pharmacists must manage cannabis dispensaries, allowing a more active role.
- More pharmacists are pursuing further education in cannabis to become cannabis specialists. Providing practitioner and patient consultation via telemedicine is a rapidly emerging opportunity for pharmacists.
- It is imperative that pharmacists use patient-centered, shared decision-making (i.e., practitioner/patient work together as a team to achieve the patient's treatment goals).

Medical Cannabis: Resource List

- *Cannabis Science & Therapeutics for Pharmacists – Online course for pharmacists on endocannabinoid system/introduction to clinical cannabis:* https://www.medicalcannabismentor.com/cannabis-science-therapeutics-for-pharmacists/
- Oberg E, Cunha JP. *"Medical Marijuana (Medical Cannabis)."* MedicineNet: https://www.medicinenet.com/medical_marijuana_medical_cannabis/article.htm (Accessed 2021)
- Bridgeman MB, Abazia DT. *"Medicinal Cannabis: History, Pharmacology, And Implications for the Acute Care Setting."* P T. 2017; 42(3):180–88.
- World Health Organization. *"The Health and Social Effects of Non-Medical Cannabis Use":* https://www.who.int/substance_abuse/publications/msbcannabis.pdf?ua=1 (Accessed 2021)
- WHO Expert Committee on Drug Dependence Pre-review: *Cannabis Plant and Cannabis Resin:* https://www.who.int/medicines/access/controlled-substances/Section5.CannabisPlant.Epidemiology.pdf?ua=1 (Accessed 2021)
- National Institutes of Health: National Center for Complementary and Integrative Health
- TRC Natural Medicines Database
- FDA Regulation of Cannabis and Cannabis-Derived Products, Including Cannabidiol (CBD)
- *Cannabinoid Clinical/Cannabinoids: Research, Effects, & Uses:* https://www.cannabinoidclinical.com/ (Accessed 2021)
- *Medical Cannabis (Medical Marijuana) Information from Dr. Dustin Sulak at Healer.com:* https://www.healer.com/ (Accessed 2021)

Cards by Swathi Varanasi and Jeanine P. Abrons

Motivational Interviewing Techniques

Technique	Description	Example
Reframing/Rephrasing	• Strategy to help patients examine their perceptions in a different manner	• If a patient says people are always bothering me about quitting smoking — you could reframe to: Those people seem to care about you a lot.
Open-ended Questions	• Questions that a patient cannot answer yes or no to, but require an explanation	• Questions that begin with who; what; when; where; how • What questions do you have?
Reflective Listening → Paraphrasing	• Listening carefully to your patients; really hearing what they are saying & allowing the patient to be the focus • Varying levels of depth may be used	• Example of statements that can be used: You are not quite sure that you are ready to make a change, but you are aware that your current behavior may negatively impact your health or it's been tough.
Restating	• Simply restate what the patient has said	• Patient says "I'm frustrated." You say: "I understand, you are frustrated."
Readiness Ruler	• Scale from 1 to 7 • Asking patient how important the change is to him or her • First establish that it is of some importance (See example) • Next, establish that there is room for improvement (See example)	• Why a 3 & not a 1? • What would it take to move you from a 3 to a 7?
Modified Envelope Technique	• Helps the patient to identify their primary reason or focus for change	• If there was one thing that would motivate you to change, what would it be?

Prepared by Jeanine P. Abrons

Empathic Communication Skills for Pharmacists

👍 Non-Verbal Communication

- Maintain appropriate level of eye contact to show your focus on the discussion.
- Sit down or kneel to speak at or below the patient's eye level to remove power dynamics.
- Respond appropriately with gestures (i.e., nodding) to show active listening.
- Lean in to show your engagement and interest in the conversation.
- Have a relaxed and good posture to set the tone and mood of the room.
- Match your facial expression to the situation or mood of the conversation.

👎 Non-Verbal Communication

- Don't yawn or limit eye contact. This may show disinterest in a conversation.
- Avoid closed body language (i.e., crossed arms, clenched fists, or slouched shoulders) as you may be viewed as defensive or difficult to approach.
- Avoid leaning back. This may appear as being too relaxed and not taking the conversation seriously.
- Be careful to not check the time with a watch/phone/clock as it may make patients feel rushed, less important, unheard, and even a burden.

Responding to Emotions
- It is inevitable in healthcare that you will encounter patients who may be overwhelmed with emotions, especially when they are trying to cope with unfavorable situations involving their health.
- Until overwhelming emotions are addressed, continuing a conversation by communicating with facts or logic may be ineffective and inappropriate.
- It is important to remember that regardless of the situation, the hurdles that people face are all relative to & dependent on their own perspectives.
- Everyone has the right to feel their emotions!
- Supporting patients through these difficult situations requires healthcare providers to take a step back to utilize their insight and empathy.
- Many different emotions (i.e., fear, regret, helplessness) can be expressed as anger or frustration. If someone appears angry or upset, do not take it personally, as they may just need someone to listen with empathy.

Card written by Theodore Nguyen and Kashelle Lockman.

Delivering Bad News

Pharmacists often share upsetting or disappointing news with patients. Examples include telling patients about unavailable medications, sharing unfavorable test results, discussing medication errors, or addressing medical encounters complicated by systemic racism or prejudices. The SPIKES acronym provides a framework to share & discuss bad news with patients and families.

\multicolumn{3}{c}{SPIKES Acronym for Breaking Bad News}		
Acronym	**Explanation**	**Example Scenario**
S	**Setting**	Ensure that you fully understand the current situation and are prepared to answer any questions that may arise. If possible, go to a private and quiet setting to avoid distractions.	• You are a pharmacist about to break the bad news to a patient that there is an unavailable prescription due to a nation-wide drug shortage. • Bring the patient to a private consult room or window distanced from others within the pharmacy.
P	**Perception**	Ask questions to get a better understanding of the patient's perspective and what they already know.	• "What did your doctor tell you about this medication?" • "How do you feel about taking this medication? . . . Tell me more . . ."
I	**Invitation**	Provide patients with a warning shot to prepare them for bad news. If appropriate, you may want to ask patients if they would like more information first.	• "Unfortunately, I have some bad news . . ." • "Can I share some disappointing news with you?"
K	**Knowledge**	When sharing knowledge, keep it concise and simple. Avoid medical jargon or providing excessive information or evidence unless requested by the patient.	• "There is a national shortage, and I do not have your medication in stock."
E	**Emotions**	Before patients can process facts and logic, they need to have their emotions addressed. *(See "Responding to Emotions" section below.)*	• Utilize the NURSE mnemonic, silence, and "I wish" statements. • "It sounds like you're very worried about your blood pressure without this medication. I am too. I wish I could guarantee we can have your medication ready for you before you run out."
S	**Summarize & Strategize**	Summarize the discussion. Explain how you will move a plan forward with the patient.	• "Since there is a shortage, I can't dispense your medication today. I will continually monitor our supplier website and the inventory of my other locations. I will call your physician to see if there is a different medication they can prescribe in the meantime. I will update you by 6 p.m. today."

Card written by Theodore Nguyen and Kashelle Lockman.

NURSE Acronym for Responding to Emotions

Acronym	Explanation		Try Saying	Avoid Saying
N	Naming the Emotion	Identify and name an emotion the patient is experiencing out loud to help validate how they feel and help you connect.	• "It looks like you might be concerned about..." • "That sounds very disappointing..." • "This seems frustrating..."	• "You must be..." • "You shouldn't be..."
U	Understanding	Verbalize how you can see the situation from their perspective. This can help you align with the patient as an ally and decreases the chance they will feel negatively judged. Unless you have experienced the same medical and social situation, avoid saying, "I understand..."	• "With everything that has happened, I can see why..."	• "I understand that you are going through..." • "I know how you feel..."
R	Respecting	Utilize statements of respect to help validate the experiences and/or challenges that patients have undergone. Avoid belittling, marginalizing, or judgmental comments.	• "You've done everything you could..." • "You have been so strong..."	• "Everyone has to deal with it..." • "Other people have it worse..." • "You should have called three days ago..."
S	Supporting	Provide comments of your support to the patient to help alleviate patient feelings of anxiety and unrest. Avoid silver-lining situations or infusing false hope.	• "This must be difficult, and our team is here to help you..." • "I will be here to help you as best I can..."	• "Don't worry, it'll be fine."
E	Exploring	Ask the patient questions to explore their emotion/situation. This may give you a better understanding of your patient and potentially enough information for a resolution.	• "Tell me more..." • "What do you think about..."	• "Okay, great." • "You must feel ___ because..." • "Anyway, let's talk about your medicine."

Card written by Theodore Nguyen and Kashelle Lockman.

Differentiating Empathy Versus Sympathy

Empathy and sympathy are commonly mistaken as synonyms as they both deal with emotions. Sympathy is often referred to as a feeling of care and concern. Empathy refers to having the ability to understand and share the emotion someone is experiencing through their unique perspective. Utilizing empathy allows for the development of a more profound connection between pharmacists and their patients, fostering a deeper level of trust. Patients may become more comfortable with sharing vital pieces of information or come to rely on the pharmacist's professional advice for shared decision making.

Empathic Statements "I wish..."	Sympathetic Statements "I'm sorry..."
• Ability to recognize and share emotions with someone. • Attempts to see the patient's unique perspective on a situation. • Requires a level of vulnerability to emotionally situate themselves with others. • Allows pharmacists to build emotional connections with patients.	• Feeling of care or concern for someone. • Simply acknowledges a negative event has occurred and prevents further exploration of the patient's experience. • This can sometimes be mistaken for pity. • Can shift focus away from the patient and family to the pharmacist's feelings.

"I Wish" Statements
Utilizing "I wish" statements allows pharmacists to connect and align with patients while acknowledging the true nature of an unfortunate situation. These statements give an opportunity for pharmacists to reveal their shared feelings for a desired outcome, even if it may not be realistic, without providing patients with false hope.

Speaking Volumes with Silence
- Effective communication involves appropriate utilization of pauses in speaking to allow time for processing information or reflecting on current emotions.
- Silence can be awkward if it is used inappropriately or with uncertainty. It may take time to master the appropriate pauses in speech.
- Silence should be used with intent. Some instances include allowing patients to think and feel after an empathic response or when sharing a moment of compassion.

Card written by Theodore Nguyen and Kashelle Lockman.

Common Problematic Phrases in Communication to Avoid

There are common phrases that can have negative connotations to patients, and that are often overlooked by providers. This can cause strain in developing rapport.

Avoid saying...	Why?	Instead, try saying...
"...withdrawal of care." "There's nothing more that can be done." "It is what it is."	This tells the patient or family that the provider is no longer able to provide any additional care—this has a connotation of futility or patient abandonment. Even if there are no life-prolonging options in therapy, we can still provide care to improve their quality of life.	"Although this may no longer be an option, we can ___ instead..."
"It's not my fault..." "It's ___'s fault..." "I'm just the messenger."	Redirecting blame is a tactic of avoidance. This does not help the patient and their current frustrations.	"I wish this hadn't happened to you, and I will do my best to help you."
"Since you are a diabetic..." "Opioid abuser/addict"	A patient is not an illness, but a whole person.	Patient-first language: "Since you have diabetes..." "Person living with diabetes" "Person living with opioid use disorder"
"Narcotic"	This is a legal, not a medical, term that can contribute to stigma and undermine the pharmacist–patient relationship.	"Opioid medication"
"Preferred pronouns"	This phrase insinuates there are other acceptable options by which to refer to a person besides their identified pronouns.	"Pronouns"
"Alcoholic" "Heroin user" "Drug addict"	Avoid using terms that elicit stigmas and negative bias and that blame people instead of acknowledging them as people who suffer from serious illnesses that need treatment.	"Alcohol use disorder" "Opioid use disorder" "Substance use disorder"
"Mentally ill"	Recognize the patient as a person with a mental illness instead of addressing them as a disorder.	"A person with mental illness"

Card written by Theodore Nguyen and Kashelle Lockman.

References
- "Quick Guides." VITALtalk. https://www.vitaltalk.org/resources/quick-guides/
- "Bridging Inequity: Understanding Patients' Experiences." VITALtalk. https://www.vitaltalk.org/guides/bridging-inequity/
- "Serious News: Breaking Bad News Using the GUIDE Tool." VITALtalk. https://www.vitaltalk.org/guides/serious-news/
- MR Hoffman. "The Sound of Silence—When There Are No Words." Jama 322, 117 (2019).
- AL Back, SM Bauer-Wu, CH Rushton, & J Halifax. "Compassionate silence in the patient-clinician encounter: A contemplative approach." J. Palliat. Med. 12, 1113–17 (2009).
- "Communication: What Do Patients Want and Need?" J Oncol Pract. 2008;4(5):249–53.
- WF Baile, R Buckman, R Lenzi, G Glober, EA Beale, & AP Kudelka. "SPIKES-A six-step protocol for delivering bad news: application to the patient with cancer." Oncologist. 2000;5(4):02–11.
- TE Quill, RM Arnold, & F Platt. "'I Wish Things Were Different': Expressing Wishes in Response to Loss, Futility, and Unrealistic Hopes." Ann. Intern. Med. 135, 551 (2001).
- JF Kelly, R Saitz, & S Wakeman. "Language, Substance Use Disorders, and Policy: The Need to Reach Consensus on an 'addiction-ary'." Alcohol. Treat. Q. 34, 116–23 (2016).

Pharmacists' Patient Care Process

Pharmacists' Patient Care Process
Pharmacists use a patient-centered approach in collaboration with other providers on the health care team to optimize patient health and medication outcomes.

Using principles of evidence-based practice, pharmacists:

Collect
The pharmacist assures the collection of the necessary subjective and objective information about the patient in order to understand the relevant medical/medication history and clinical status of the patient.

Assess
The pharmacist assesses the information collected and analyzes the clinical effects of the patient's therapy in the context of the patient's overall health goals in order to indentify and prioritize problems and achieve optimal care.

Plan
The pharmacist develops an individualized patient-centered care plan, in collaboration with other health care professionals and the patient or caregiver that is evidence based and cost effective.

Implement
The pharmacist implements the care plan in collaboration with other health care professionals and the patient or caregiver.

Follow-up: Monitor and Evaluate
The pharmacist monitors and evaluates the effectiveness of the care plan and modifies the plan in collaboration with other health care professionals and the patient or caregiver as needed.

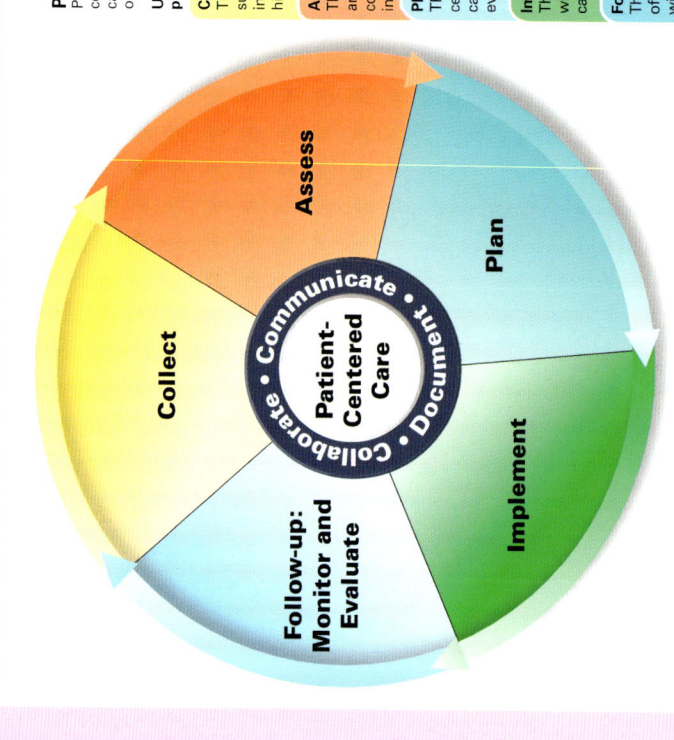

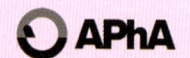

Source: *Joint Commission of Pharmacy Practitioners, 2014*

Pharmacists' Patient Care Process *(continued)*

The Patient
- When completing the "Collect" step, consider the purpose of the patient workup:
  - Is it to present to an interdisciplinary team or pharmacist?
  - Is it to identify interventions?
  - What are the expectations for the setting and situation?
- Some settings/situations you may need less of this information, while in others you may need more.
- The following are the portions of the Pharmacist Patient Care Process associated with each step: Steps 1 and 2 represent the "Collect" portion; Steps 3 to 6 represent the "Assess" portion; Steps 7 and 8 represent the "Plan" portion; Step 9 represents the "Implement" portion; Step 10 represents the "Follow-up: Monitor and Evaluate" portion.

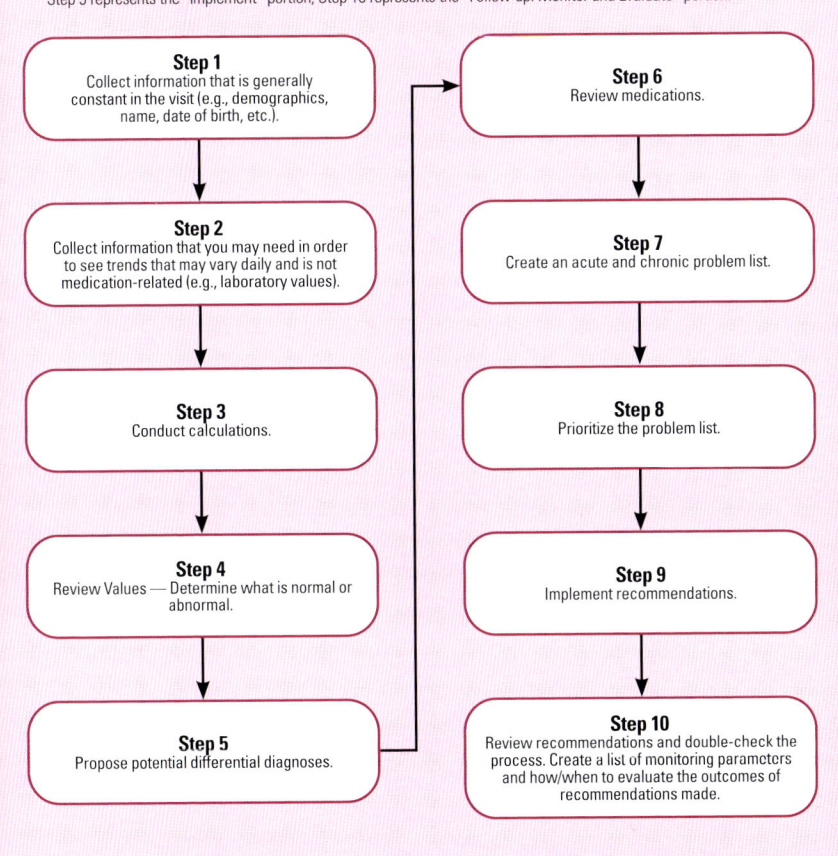

Step 1
Collect information that is generally constant in the visit (e.g., demographics, name, date of birth, etc.).

Step 2
Collect information that you may need in order to see trends that may vary daily and is not medication-related (e.g., laboratory values).

Step 3
Conduct calculations.

Step 4
Review Values — Determine what is normal or abnormal.

Step 5
Propose potential differential diagnoses.

Step 6
Review medications.

Step 7
Create an acute and chronic problem list.

Step 8
Prioritize the problem list.

Step 9
Implement recommendations.

Step 10
Review recommendations and double-check the process. Create a list of monitoring parameters and how/when to evaluate the outcomes of recommendations made.

Choosing Your Counseling Points

Things to Remember

Things to remember when counseling:
☐ Tailor counseling to the needs of your specific patient (i.e., age, breast-feeding, pregnant, etc.). Content should be individualized to enhance the usefulness to your patient.
☐ Patient's health literacy or the ability to obtain, process, & understand basic information varies widely. ○ *Health literacy is the degree to which individuals have capacity to obtain, process, & understand basic health information & services needed to make appropriate health decisions.* • *This can include numeracy (understanding numbers, calculations, measurements).* • *This can include basic literacy (reading, writing, speaking, & computing/solving problems).* • *This is dependent on communication skills, lay/professional knowledge, culture, demands of healthcare, & demands of the situation.* ○ *Only 12% of adults have proficient health literacy.*
☐ Simplify both written & verbal communication using clear language, nonmedical terms, & easy-to-read formats; be specific (e.g., timing).
☐ Organize information logically. Focus & list three to five most important "need-to-know" points with the most important points first.
☐ Break complex information into understandable chunks.
☐ Use the medication bottle while counseling to show the patient where to find information on the label.
☐ Use the medication leaflet & circle important information. Write additional notes to help a patient remember information when they get home. ○ *If writing information, take care to ensure readability. Text should be written at the 6th-grade reading level.*
☐ Reinforce information to ensure retention. ○ *Utilize the teach-back method or stop after each key point and allow the patient to ask questions.*
☐ Consider whether translation services are needed and whether print information should be provided in another language to ensure understanding of content.

Select References: (Accessed 2021)
1. Health Literacy: https://health.gov/communication/literacy/quickguide/factsbasic.htm
2. https://nnlm.gov/initiatives/topics/health-literacy
3. Readability: https://www.wyliecomm.com/2019/03/us-literacy-rate/ & http://www.clearlanguagegroup.com/readability/

Cards by Angela Wojtczak and Jeanine P. Abrons

Choosing Your Counseling Points *(continued)*

Medication-Specific Guidance

Medication-Specific Counseling
☐ Name of the medication: brand & generic
☐ Have you taken this medication before? ○ *Remember to ask what they recall if they have taken the medication before & adjust counseling points to either correct discrepancies or fill in pieces of knowledge that they've forgotten.* ○ *Let the patient know if there has been a manufacturer or appearance change.*
☐ Indication: Ask, "What could you use the medication for? ○ *For new prescriptions, first ask: "What did the healthcare provider tell you this was for?"*
☐ Dose (i.e., amount), route (i.e., how the medication is taken), & frequency (i.e., how often the medication is taken)
☐ Provide administration tips: ○ *With/without food* ○ *Does it require separation from other medications or vitamins/supplements?* ○ *Specific timing*
☐ Discuss with the patient what to do: ○ *A missed dose occurs* ○ *When to stop the medication (if at all), acute versus chronic use* ○ *If monitoring (if laboratory work) is needed, when should this be done; who will do the monitoring & how should it be scheduled/coordinated?* ○ *When the next follow up (next appointment) should occur & what to report at this time*
☐ Discuss with the patient what to expect: ○ *Medication onset & duration of effect i.e., How long will it take to start working? How long should it work?* ○ *How to know if the medication is working* ○ *What to expect with adverse effects or reactions—Present adverse effects as being common (> 10 to 15%) (e.g., sun-sensitivity), notable, & rare, but serious side effects (e.g., blackbox warnings such as hepatotoxicity)* ○ *Highlight possible interactions with medications, vitamins, & supplements, alcohol, & foods (e.g., grapefruit). Brainstorm what the patient can do to minimize these interactions (e.g., spacing out dosing; avoidance). If interactions cannot be avoided, discuss what the impact to other medications may be & what to monitor for.*

Cards by Angela Wojtczak and Jeanine P. Abrons.

Choosing Your Counseling Points *(continued)*

Other Counseling Items

General Counseling
☐ Explain the importance of adherence and discuss strategies that can increase adherence. 　○ *Examples: Benefits of daily routines, pill boxes, assistance from a family member/friend, calendars, alarms, or lists. Do not assume adherence is due to not remembering.*
☐ Consider Social Determinants of Health 　○ *Does the patient have insurance? Has there been a change of employment/living situation? Can the patient afford the medication? Are there barriers in time & transportation to get the medication?*
☐ Proper storage & disposal—unique aspects
☐ Number of refills & how to obtain a refill
☐ Who to contact in case of question/concern/adverse drug effects or reactions

How to Improve Health Literacy & Patient Understanding
☐ Use short, easy words; without jargon 　○ *Not everyone has the same vocabulary level* 　○ *Words with less syllables are easier to understand*
☐ Shorten your sentences or break up large sentences
☐ Take out unnecessary adjectives or adverbs
☐ Refrain from using jargon or medical vocabulary. Also, consider defining words that may be more difficult to understand.
☐ Use simple fonts 　○ *Example:* Times New Roman, Arial, or Helvetica
☐ Use illustrations, pictures, graphs, & different shading to enhance appeal of your materials & the reader's attention.
☐ Highlight important points by bolding the content.
☐ Consider use of readability formulas (e.g., Flesch-Kinkaid Reading Ease or Grade Level, Gunning Fog Scores, Smog Index)

Cards by Angela Wojtczak and Jeanine P. Abrons; updated by Jeanine P. Abrons.